Dr Jane McCartney is a chartered psychologist
specialising in overeating issues.

STOP
OVEREATING

The 28-day plan
to end emotional eating

Dr Jane McCartney

Vermilion
LONDON

1 3 5 7 9 10 8 6 4 2

First published in 2014 by Vermilion, an imprint of Ebury Publishing
A Random House Group company

The Random House Group Limited Reg. No. 954009

Addresses for companies within the Random House Group can be found at
www.randomhouse.co.uk

The Random House Group Limited supports the Forest Stewardship
Council® (FSC®), the leading international forest-certification organisation.
Our books carrying the FSC label are printed on FSC®-certified paper. FSC is
the only forest-certification scheme supported by the leading environmental
organisations, including Greenpeace. Our paper procurement policy can
be found at www.randomhouse.co.uk/environment

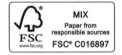

Designed and set by seagulls.net

Printed in the UK by CPI Group (UK) Ltd, Croydon, CR0 4YY

ISBN 9780091954994

To buy books by your favourite authors and register for offers visit
www.randomhouse.co.uk

To my wonderful family, Steve, Joe, Harvey and Elsa. Thanks for all your valued support, welcome encouragement and endless recipe tastings.

CONTENTS

contents

Introduction   1

**Session 1/Week1: Understanding the Emotional
Chain of Events**   9
Part 1: The Emotional Trigger   12
Part 2: The Experienced Emotion   27
Part 3: The Negative Emotional Message and Your   37
        Relationships

Session 2/Week 2: Me and Food – What Happened?   65
Part 1: Your Relationship with Food   68
Part 2: Habits, Addictions and Pre-occupations   82
        with Food
Part 3: The Beliefs of an Emotional Eater   91

Session 3/Week 3: Start to Stop   103
Part 1: The Mini Moment Intervention   105
Part 2: The Maxi Effect Analysis   117
Part 3: Challenging   138

Session 4/Week 4: Moving Beyond Emotional Eating   155
Part 1: Saboteurs   157
Part 2: FOMO – The Fear of Missing Out   172
Part 3: Allowance Days   178

28-day Eating Plan   183

Conclusion   265
Acknowledgements   269
Index   271

introduction

'Over and over again I would go on this diet or that eating programme and at first I'd be doing really well. Then something or other would happen and I'd find it so utterly disheartening and demotivating that all that effort would be out of the window in a flash. I could never say what it was in particular – little things, big things, I believe it's called life – and no matter what my good intentions were, I always seemed to end up turning to food to cope.'

If this sounds familiar to you, perhaps you are one of the many serial but unsuccessful dieters who, despite your genuine best efforts, either stay overweight or just keep piling on the pounds. You are stuck in a never-ending cycle of being really motivated to lose weight, starting the diet, losing a bit of weight, something happening, the diet failing, the weight going back on and moving on to yet another diet.

So why does this happen? Well, through no fault of your own you are probably like over 70 per cent of people who struggle with their weight: you are an emotional eater. You understand that eating high-calorie, high-fat and sugar-loaded foods is keeping you overweight, but somehow you just can't seem to resist eating them when you feel under emotional strain.

It is highly unlikely that you suddenly became an emotional eater as an adult or teenager; the emotional groundwork was already in place just waiting for the opportunity to emerge. If you do genuinely think that you have only recently become an emotional eater, chances are it has probably been building up for years and recently some external emotional trigger has set it off. The habit of emotional eating is amazingly quick to learn and, like lots of habits, once established it is very hard to break. The principle of *Stop Overeating* is for you to learn to separate your emotions, and how they subsequently make you feel about yourself, away from food so you will not end up eating when an upsetting or distressing situation or encounter occurs.

With the help of this book, you will at last be able to understand, overcome and manage your emotionally driven eating and achieve your goal to lose weight once and for all. You will equip yourself with the psychological tools you need to reach the very best position to undertake a diet, accomplish your weight-loss plan and, crucially, maintain the weight loss at the end of it.

Throughout my career as a qualified psychologist and therapist I have successfully helped many people understand and challenge the psychological and emotional reasons for turning to food. Through weekly one-to-one sessions, clients explore and challenge their emotional need to eat, including what underlies it, who provokes it and what their unconscious eating patterns and habits around emotional eating are. Now in this easy-to-follow book, you too can gain the benefits of a dedicated therapy course.

When it comes to dieting and weight loss, your emotions are going to play a very important role in your success, whether you are an emotional eater or not. For example, you could be affected by how you feel about yourself for being overweight to begin with, or how you feel about denying yourself certain foods. Other people's attitudes towards you are important, not just as someone who is overweight, but also more generally – are you valued and treated fairly? Do your opinions matter? These are just some of the many psychological aspects that you will address so that you can reach your target weight once and for all.

Often, the 'eat less, do more'-type diet books do not take these considerations into account. They usually only ever focus on your calorie intake and completely overlook the psychological side of things, which to me is a bit like changing the tyres on a broken car when it is the engine that needs far more attention.

As well as being a qualified psychologist and therapist, I was also an emotional eater and serial dieter myself. Believe me, I know the emotional pitfalls, the irritations, the highs and lows of losing weight, not losing weight or putting on weight when you have been working so hard to lose it. In other words I really know how you feel. I know what it is like to have to diet and find it really difficult to fight your emotions to stop yourself eating the contents of the fridge when something upsetting happens. My professional and personal experiences are combined in this book to help you overcome your emotional eating, as I have done.

How to Use this Book

Stop Overeating is specifically designed to give you a straightforward, focused approach so you can gain a clear understanding of the causes of your emotional eating.

The book is divided into four main chapters, which replicate a course of weekly one-to-one therapy sessions. In each chapter you will start to work out what has gone on, and continues to go on, in your life to gain some psychological order and emotional control. This will help you make sense of your feelings so you will be in a mentally strong position to reach your desired weight loss. Aim to work through one chapter per week for four weeks.

The four sessions ißn the book are:

1. Understanding the Emotional Chain of Events
In this session you will explore what happens to you psychologically and emotionally each time an upsetting and distressing situation or encounter happens to you.

2. Me and Food, What Happened?
In this session you will examine the history of your poor relationship with food and the **habits, addictions** and **pre-occupations** that have been damaging your weight-loss attempts. You'll also start to challenge your long-held **beliefs** about being an emotional eater in this second session.

3. Start to Stop

Here you will learn specific long- and short-term psychological techniques to manage and stop your emotional
eating both now and in the future. You will learn how
to effectually and accurately **challenge** any unwelcome
emotional messages you receive.

4. Moving Beyond Emotional Eating

In this final session you will explore and examine those
often-unrecognised features of your life that may impede or
stop your weight-loss and diet plans, including **saboteurs,
FOMO,** (Fear Of Missing Out) and **allowance days.**

As in traditional one-to-one therapy, each session builds
on the discoveries, information and observations from the
previous weeks. By the end of your sessions you will have
a comprehensive and new understanding of all the factors
in your life that have been impacting and fuelling your
particular style of emotional eating. And, most importantly,
you will have the psychological tools and know-how to do
something about them.

Throughout the book you will find very simple, quick
and straightforward therapy exercises for you to do. These
follow the principles and type of questions and exercises
you would have in a one-to-one therapy situation. I have
designed these exercises to help you gather important
information and observations about what underlies your
emotional eating. This may be a situation or it could be
an individual who is causing you emotional distress. Once

you get into the routine of doing the exercises they will take only a few seconds to do. Absolutely no one else need know that you are doing the exercises if you do not want them to.

It would be ideal to complete all the parts of each individual session in its allotted week. If this is not practical or feels too overwhelming, it is fine to take them at a pace that suits you. You might find doing the exercises emotionally challenging, but the fact that you have bought this book demonstrates that you are already on your way to doing something about your emotional eating and losing weight. Keep persevering and you will stay on track.

Case Studies

To support you through the sessions in *Stop Overeating*, we will follow the stories of three people – Kate, Frank and Linda – who are working through the plan.

Kate

Kate is a classic **comforter**. Whenever she has any situation or encounter with someone in her life which causes her emotional upset, Kate will instantly and habitually turn to food to comfort herself.

Frank

Frank is a **suppressor**. He depends on using food as a means of supressing, concealing and diverting himself from his unwanted emotions.

Linda

Linda is a typical **punisher**. She is pre-occupied with using food to castigate and rebuke herself for her perceived failures or stupidity when she experiences an emotionally provoking situation or encounter.

Perhaps you can recognise some familiar traits and routines in your own emotional eating. Does Kate's need for comfort from food seem familiar to you? Like Frank, do you use food to suppress or divert yourself away from the destructive and harmful message your emotions are telling you? Or do you recognise Linda's use of food as a form of punishment when you find the negative messages from your emotions too much to deal with? Maybe you find that food and eating offer a complex combination of comfort, suppression and punishment when something provoking happens and ignites unwelcome thoughts and feelings.

They say that knowledge is power, and the more under-standing you can gain about your reasons for emotional eating, the better you will be able to combat them.

The 28-day Eating Plan

Also included in this book is a 28-day Eating Plan. The plan is designed to complement the therapy chapters and help you to stay on track. You'll find tasty ideas for breakfast, lunch, dinner and even desserts that will keep you feeling full and satisfied. There are over 40 delicious recipes to try – you might be surprised at what you can eat while still keeping an eye on your weight!

Many of my clients find it really useful to follow the eating plan as it saves them having to think too long and hard about what they are going to eat during their psychological therapy, which allows them to focus on processing their emotional findings.

It's also great to get a good headstart in losing weight. If you follow the plan for 28 days, you will find it so much easier to carry on afterwards. You may want to repeat the menu plan for another 28 days (it has been designed to offer a good variety of meals so you will not get bored). Alternatively, you may wish to devise your own healthy meals. Either way, once you have begun to lose weight, you will be much more motivated to continue until you reach your desired weight.

I wish you every success in following the *Stop Overeating* plan. So many people have found that having a proper psychological tool to support their weight loss has been the key thing missing through all their years of yo-yo, frustrating and endless dieting. This is your chance to take control of your eating habits for good to turn your life and your health around.

session 1 / week 1

Understanding the Emotional Chain of Events

Introduction

In this first week of the *Stop Overeating* plan, you are going to look in detail at three aspects of emotional eating that are keeping you both overweight and a disillusioned and unsuccessful dieter. The emotional chain of events is what happens each and every time you experience an upsetting or distressing situation or encounter that leads to an episode of overeating. It is a rapid set of psychological emotional reactions formed of:

1. An **emotional trigger** – the big, little and anything-in-between things which happen to you on a daily basis and cause you emotional upset.
2. The **experienced emotion** – the specific and very personal emotions caused by the trigger event.
3. The **negative emotional messages** – the resulting emotional messages that you receive.

Emotional eating often happens to you so quickly that the situation or encounter somehow becomes an accepted part of the whole process, but it is crucial that you take the time to properly identify your external triggers. If you can start to build up an awareness of the types of situations, encounters or memories that cause your emotional eating, they will not always have the devastating physical and psychological effect on you that they have done up until now.

The second part of the emotional eating chain of events is your internal emotional response: the experienced emotions you feel each time something happens in your life to upset you. It is important to accurately identify the emotions so you can recognise any themes, clusters or patterns.

These specific unwanted internal emotions in turn send upsetting, distressing negative emotional messages to you, which is the third part of your focus in this first session. The negative emotional messages are the reason you become an emotional eater. You find these negative messages so intolerable, unwelcome and damaging that over the years you will have sought comfort with food, or you will use food to suppress or restrain the negative message in some way. You may also use food as a form of punishment because you agree with the negative message – that you are worthless, not good enough, unlovable and so on. You may do just one of these, a combination of them or, as with a lot of emotional eaters, all three. In the investigation into the negative emotional message you will also make your first detailed analysis of the relationships in your life which are likely to be big contributors to your emotional eating.

As *Stop Overeating* is mirroring a traditional one-to-one therapy model, try to undertake all the parts of each individual session in one week, and as close to each other as possible. Read through the entire session first to familiarise yourself with what you need to do, then do the Backward Step Technique exercise followed by the Emotion Identifier exercise and the Statement of Feelings exercise. Ideally, you will complete all the exercises in one go. It may seem like a lot at first but once you are familiar with the exercises you can start to put them all together for the emotionally provoking situations and encounters you then experience. If you feel a little overwhelmed at any point it is okay to slow down or take a breather for a short while and pick up where you left off later.

It is great that you want to do something positive about losing weight. It will be a major psychological undertaking and this may seem like a tall order right now, because you are in the habit of trying to deal with what happens to you emotionally with food. It will be hard work, but I have seen many people successfully lose weight using a psychological approach together with the 28-day Eating Plan. So, let's get started …

Part 1
The Emotional Trigger

Throughout this book you will be following three different people – Kate, Frank and Linda – as they undertake the four weeks of the *Stop Overeating* plan to manage their long-standing emotional eating problems. In this first session their stories will show what they identified as contributors to their most recent episode of emotional eating. Perhaps you will find yourself nodding in agreement.

In this part of the session you are going to be examining and starting to analyse the chain of events that makes you an emotional eater. You will learn how to identify, name and begin to predict the external emotion-triggering situations and encounters in your life which may be behind your overeating.

The emotional chain of events is set off by an upsetting or disturbing emotional trigger. It is this trigger which you will need to clearly identify in order to do something about it. The trigger may be something in the here and now, such as missing the bus or an argument with your partner. Or it could be persistent long-term issues, like dysfunctional family relationships or work problems.

Knowing how to uncover and identify what is really causing your emotional eating will be the very best start to stopping it. Right now you may think it sounds unnecessary to have a dedicated process to identify what upsets and distresses you. However, this step is vital because eventually you will learn how to stop your emotional eating right at the beginning of an upsetting situation before any overeating harm is done, in other words before you eat anything which is damaging to your weight loss.

Finding Out What's Going On

When you emotionally eat, what generally happens is that you get caught up in the whole emotional chain of events. The actual starting point, the external trigger, can somehow get completely lost and forgotten in the process. But the problem is that if the emotional triggers are not properly identified, there is then nothing to stop them from resurfacing the next time and the time after that, and you will simply carry on being upset and distressed and emotionally eating.

Some emotional eaters, who get so involved and caught up in the sourcing, buying and actual eating of the food itself, honestly cannot remember any specific triggers which upset them in the first place. If prompted, perhaps they could recollect some vague incident or event to link with an episode of emotional eating. However, for others, the finite detail of the situation or encounter is painfully etched on their consciousness and merely the slightest recall of it can have them reaching for food to deal with it all over again.

Either way something happens which ultimately leads to emotional eating in order to cope with the intolerable and unwelcome negative emotional messages the trigger provokes. Remember, the cause of your emotional eating is how you feel about yourself at any one time. So it is crucial to get a clear and accurate understanding of the external factors that affect how you feel in order to become consciously aware of their potential psychological damage – and to eventually be able to stop them from harming you.

Upsetting things are going to happen in your life, they do to everyone, but once you learn how to tolerate them you can learn to manage and stop your emotional eating. You are capable of controlling how you react in a way that is much less self-destructive than overeating, which you will learn how to do in the third session, Start to Stop (see page 103). After what is probably a lifetime of reaching for the biscuits or crisps to cope, you have understandably forgotten what to do instead. It may seem daunting, but there is no reason why you cannot succeed.

Going Back to Help Go Forward

Over the many years of providing therapy to people who want to lose weight, and for my own personal use, I have devised and developed a number of very quick and straightforward exercises to help discover what is really going on emotionally. The first is the very simple Backward Step Technique (see page 16) to uncover the triggers in your life which ultimately contribute to your eventual eating, weight gain and dieting failures.

In the Backward Step Technique you give yourself space to focus on the main causes of your emotional eating. As you become more familiar with this particular technique you will start to understand what is most relevant for you in an episode of emotional eating. For instance you may think that the pressure of your work is the sole cause of you reaching for the chocolate biscuits throughout the day. However, it could be just as much your home and family dynamics or relationship issues which are causing and contributing to your overeating. As these are quite often persistent longer-term problems, which have become a subconsciously accepted part of your life, their contribution and significance to your emotional eating can be overlooked and unacknowledged, and therefore dangerously unchallenged and allowed to continue.

I devised the Backward Step Technique so you could start thinking honestly about what, and who, has caused your emotional eating in a detailed and analytical way, rather than taking everything on and being completely overwhelmed. In the Backward Step Technique you are going to consider just five things which, separately or combined, pushed you to the point of your most recent episode of emotional eating.

Your Flight of Stairs

Having or wanting to emotionally eat is a little bit like being on the top step of a short flight of stairs, where the top step represents your emotional eating episode. In this exercise you are going to think about and consider your most recent episode of emotional eating. You cannot just take the episode as a standalone event; lots of other things will be associated with it. It is not just going to be *'I had a bad journey to work so I had two doughnuts and a large hot chocolate the moment I got to my desk'*. Lots of other events will be contributing to it: the children not getting up ready for school, not charging your mobile phone, still not talking to your brother after falling out six years ago. It is anything at all which then goes on to impact negatively on how you feel about yourself, both during and sometime after the event, which is important to identify. You need to start looking at what you consider to be the significant contributory factors which led up to your emotional eating so you can do something about them.

Using this simple Backward Step Technique is a very straightforward and effective way of uncovering your emotional triggers. It is called the Backward Step Technique because you will take a detailed reverse look at the most recent contributors to your latest episode of emotional eating.

The Backward Step Technique

In one-to-one therapy you have your own dedicated space to discuss what has been happening to you. *Stop Overeating* is no different so make sure you have proper time, quiet and space to really think about things; this is your time to concentrate on yourself.

Step One

For this first exercise, set aside some time in your day and try to find a quiet place. It is best to write everything down – it will be needed for the other exercises in this session. You could keep notes of your thoughts and findings on your phone, or in an email to yourself – anything which suits you is fine. Some people find it helpful to draw some very basic steps and then fill them in with the triggering situations.

Step Two

Think about a recent episode when you have emotionally eaten, or when you have had that familiar urge to eat because of how you feel and not because of genuine physical hunger. Write down the episode itself as your 'top step'. Then, for the Backward Step Technique, you take a step backwards or down on your staircase and consider one specific event that led you to the top step. Then repeat this and take a step backwards four more times. The five most significant contributors do not have to be in a specific order, but people usually find it quite useful to think of the incident which happened closest in time to the emotional eating to start with. Often when I have done this exercise with clients they have found it useful to physically step backwards. It does not have to be any great movement and can be done very discreetly. It just helps some people to focus on the emotional triggers.

Step Three

You should now have six 'steps' on your staircase – your top step is the emotional eating situation, then up to five causes that led to the situation. If you are struggling to fill in all five steps, it is fine to leave it with as many as you have thought and made a note of. If something comes up later which you feel is valid, you can add it in or make a note of it for the next time you do the Backward Step Technique.

Do not take too long to do this exercise; you want your response and thoughts to be as instinctive and unmodified as possible. Once you get into the habit of doing this, you will be able to complete the technique without having to write things down. It is important to keep going on this exercise, even if you find it challenging. Take a short breather if you need to, but this is your first chance to begin to see what makes you an emotional eater, so stay with it.

Case Study: Kate

Kate knew she needed help after an incident at her work. A colleague had brought in a huge cake to share in the office but did not offer any to Kate. Kate said everyone else was given some cake and, even though someone eventually brought some over for her, Kate said she felt abandoned, ignored, rejected and really upset by the whole incident. At lunchtime Kate threw away her salad and went out to buy the biggest cream cake she could find. She spent her whole lunchtime sitting alone on a bench eating it all by herself. Kate said this was by no means the first time something similar had happened both at work and in other aspects of her life. Kate felt eating the cake by herself was the final indication that she needed to address her out-of-control emotional overeating.

'So there I was, having eaten the whole cream cake by myself, my top step. I couldn't stop myself – I had to finish the whole thing. When I thought about the five things that had got me to that the point, the first thing/step that came to mind as a potential cause was the spiteful colleague. I was brought in to do her job two years previously and she'd never particularly liked me, never even spoken to me really. But it wasn't just that. I was worried about my relationship with my new husband – the second step. We've been married six months and, when I'd told him about things like this in the past, I wasn't sure he really listened or understood what I was saying. Which led to the next step backwards – number three on my list – if my own husband doesn't understand me how can I expect anyone else to? It made me feel really lonely and insecure. I saw the fourth step as having to go and see my parents soon. It was their 30th wedding anniversary party, which I spent ages helping to organise, but I wasn't really looking forward to it. Visiting

> my parents for their anniversary was the fourth step, but
> it was also linked to the final step of what I think made
> me emotionally eat the cake that lunchtime and why I
> habitually emotionally overeat, and have done throughout
> my life – my older sister, Emma. She still lives at home
> with Mum and Dad and has got plenty of her own issues
> with food. In fact she's the complete opposite to me:
> skinny, underweight and a fussy eater. Emma had sent
> me one of her demanding texts saying how I'd left her
> to do all the work for Mum and Dad's anniversary, which
> was not true. The tone and attitude of her texts, calls
> and emails upset me and made me feel really bad about
> myself for not doing enough. Practically every time I hear
> from Emma, I want to go straight to the bakery or cake
> shop afterwards.'

When you start identifying all the potential causes of your emotional eating, it can be difficult to stop – that is why for the exercise you limit yourself to five triggering steps each time. You need enough so you can see what has contributed to a particular episode of emotional eating, but not so many that you end up with an endless and exhaustive list of issues in your life, which could quickly lead to a '*What's the point?*' moment. Many of the triggers will cross over to other episodes of emotional eating. Getting a clear idea of the actual contributors to your emotional eating is going to be essential in giving you the control to stop it. Like all the exercises in *Stop Overeating*, there is no right or wrong answer, it is just a way for you to see what is going on for you psychologically that ends up with eating and weight gain.

Case Study: Frank

Frank came for help after he had a falling out with his girlfriend over money in general, and specifically about not being able to afford a party for their six-year-old twin boys' forthcoming birthday. Frank says he has always had difficulties talking about situations like this – it makes him feel uncomfortable and inadequate, but he feels if he does not do something now he never will. After their latest row, Frank drove straight to the supermarket and bought as much junk food as he could afford, as he often does, and then sat in the car park eating it all until he felt he could face going home again.

'I find it really hard to go back and think about all the things that got me in to the position of binging on junk food in the supermarket car park. Afterwards I always just want to forget about it all – the wasted money, the row and the shame of what I've done. But I know that if I'm ever going to do something about my emotional eating, I'm going to have to make myself start thinking about what causes it in the first place. The first thing on my steps list is the relationship with my girlfriend. We've got six-year-old twin boys, which I appreciate takes up a lot of her time, and she's got her own psychological problems, she suffers from depression and low mood quite a bit. The second step on my list is that I've never had that many friends, and, because I never have the

*money, and the boys take up so much time, I feel quite
isolated. The third step is that not having enough money
makes me feel unable to provide for my family, which
is always very upsetting. I work in IT, but there's not
been much work around lately. Next step – number
four – when I went to the supermarket to binge I also
had to get some petrol, but I couldn't get the petrol cap
off. I had to ask the bloke next to me for help and, even
though we were having a laugh about it, deep down it
was so humiliating. The fifth and final step, and this is
a constant issue, at nearly 20 stone my health is really
suffering, which of course makes me really worried that
I won't be around for the twins in the future.'*

It would be useful, even at this first stage of analysing
your emotional chain of events, to identify any themes,
situations or people from your Backward Step Technique
exercise which you feel contribute to your emotional eating.
Perhaps when you have to do a specific job or task that you
find starts off an emotional chain of events. Or perhaps
having to deal with the same people in your life all the time
triggers your emotional eating over and over again.

Case Study: Linda

Linda started to see me because she felt her intake
of food and subsequent weight gain was increasing
almost daily. She said she felt she was becoming almost
obsessed by eating as a way of coping with everything
upsetting in her life, but knew eating was not working

because she still had problems and was just now more overweight than ever. Linda said rarely a day would go by when she did not find herself in the kitchen with empty bottles of cola in the recycling and empty family-sized crisp and biscuits packets around her. Linda has a long-term partner, Rob, an unemployed music producer, so all the family income is left to her. They have one child, a 12-year-old son, Jamie, whose behaviour at school and home is increasingly problematic. Linda gets no support or input from Rob, who says he likes to be available if a producing job comes up, and needs to spend time networking. He is rarely at home and spends very little, if any, time with Jamie.

'When I did the Backward Step Technique exercise I knew exactly what the first step of my latest episode of emotional eating was. Last night I'd just got back from Jamie's parents' evening. I'd been told about his bad behaviour at school and not-so-subtle questions had been asked about my parenting abilities. As soon as I got home I went straight to the fridge and stayed there for the rest of the night stuffing whatever I could find into my mouth, none of which I even really tasted, let alone enjoyed. With each mouthful and with every pound I gain I'm reminding myself what a useless and rubbish mum I am. My relationship with Rob, my long-term partner, is the second step – it has always caused me to emotionally eat. Although he's not physically abusive, he is quite verbally abusive and intimidating, and I can see Jamie following his example, being dismissive and hostile to *me. My third step is work, which is causing me anxieties. It's a small catering company which has been struggling for a few years. I do the admin, and increasingly I've been doing a bit of unpaid overtime because of cash flow problems. I'm trying to help the owners as much as possible, which I feel I have to do as I've been the only regular wage earner at home for years and don't want to jeopardise it. The fourth step would be my dad, who's not very well. He moved close to us a couple of years ago so I could look after him. He says I'm stupid for working for nothing, even when I try to explain they've been a really good family to work for. Dad complains that my work takes me away from home and everything I have to do there and from him too much. The fifth step is that I've just always felt a useless person, because I don't do enough for everyone – Rob, Jamie and Dad. If I had better qualifications then I'd have a better job and then Dad and Rob would be less critical and Jamie wouldn't be following their example.'*

Linda, like a lot of emotional eaters, has essentially had a lifetime of being told how rubbish she is at everything, which, as you might expect, has had an enormous emotional effect on her, as it would on absolutely anyone. It is really important to point out at this early stage that just because you feel a certain way about yourself, and perhaps like Linda you have people around you who promote that idea of yourself for various reasons, it does not make it in any way correct, accurate or reflective of the real you. Linda is being honest about what she feels starts her emotional eating. She is doing something about it now and facing up to her fears.

By undertaking an initial Backward Step Technique exercise Kate, Frank and Linda are starting to think about their eating habits, which after a lifetime of overeating is a really great start. What they and you are doing by properly uncovering the causes of your emotional eating is difficult and challenging. As I often say to my clients, make sure you give yourself some kind of acknowledgement for your achievement, even if it is just a metaphorical pat on the back for the hard work and effort you have put in.

Our case studies have used this exercise to help them start to uncover some really useful information that highlights some of the triggers and causes – their Backward Steps – to an episode of emotional eating. This begins to introduce an element of control over their eating, which they had thought disappeared long ago. It will take time, but Kate, Frank and Linda have begun the journey to address, manage and stop their own particular type of emotional eating, even at this early stage in the programme.

The Backward Step Technique exercise allows you to start doing something about your emotional eating. For most emotional eaters it all happens so frequently that the original trigger itself, as a standalone feature, often barely registers. Or maybe it is too psychologically painful to properly identify the real triggers and reasons for your emotional eating because you are fearful of change, or perhaps things are never changing for you. Like anything troubling or problematic in your life, the original triggering causes will have to be identified and eventually fixed and dealt with so the damage stops. If you had a leak in your home each time it rained, eventually you would have to investigate the initial source of the leak and deal with it. The problem is not going to go away by itself and it will just keep dripping and causing damage if left untreated. It is exactly the same with your emotional eating: by identifying the original source and causes of it, you will be starting to fix it, so you do not have to then unconsciously and mindlessly carry on emotionally eating. Understanding all of the triggers and causes is just the first essential part of stopping emotional eating for good.

If you follow the guidance in *Stop Overeating* you will at long last start to make a real difference to your future weight. Remember that using food to deal with your problems is a very well-established way of life for most emotional eaters so it will not be easy to undo and re-learn patterns of behaviour, but you are now well and truly on the path towards stopping yourself from being an emotional eater. If you have also started the 28-day Eating Plan you are going to be putting yourself in the very best position both physically and psychologically to lose weight.

Part 2
The Experienced Emotion

> ### Case Study: Hannah
>
> *'Every time I see or meet up with my mother I always end up gorging non-stop for at least a week after. I'm over 17 stone now, and my weight only ever seems to go one way. Nothing I do for my mother is right. It's moan, criticise, pick fault, question and dismiss even my simplest decision. But I feel I do have to see her, she doesn't have anyone else. I know there's a connection between seeing her and my continual weight gain, only I'm not sure exactly what and why it is.'*

As Hannah says, she understands that one of her biggest emotional triggers is seeing her mother, but Hannah does not understand the psychological details of why meeting with her mother results in emotional overeating to the extent it does. Hannah has yet to identify her actual and individual internal emotional responses to these encounters. She knows the trigger is her mother but not how the trigger and her responses are linked psychologically to cause her emotional eating. And because she does not know, her emotional eating carries on.

Emotions

In this second part of the session you are going to continue analysing the emotional chain of events to identify and explore some of the emotions that the triggers set off. It is these experienced and unwelcome emotions themselves – the second part of the emotional chain of events – that prompt the third and final part of the chain – the negative emotional messages you receive about yourself. Remember it is these negative emotional messages which you find so intolerable and uncomfortable that food is sought to deal with them.

In this part of this session you will be naming the actual, and probably familiar, emotions you feel and experience in order to understand and eventually challenge the negative message these emotions send. You may find that you have been attributing the wrong emotions to the triggering incident. Different emotions will have different negative emotional messages. To successfully challenge the truthfulness and validity of the messages, you must accurately know which ones are generated by specific situations and encounters.

Often, as with Hannah, the emotions you experience as a response to the emotional trigger – in her case seeing her mother – are automatic, unconscious and involuntary, so of course it is difficult to have any control over them. It is important to note that this response is often a learnt subconscious reaction to any emotive triggering event which has been psychologically put in place and developed over many years of upsetting experiences. Hannah has learnt that the only, but very unsatisfactory, way of dealing with her meetings with her mother is by eating. Hannah does not yet understand what goes on between experiencing the actual emotions and receiving the highly damaging negative emotional message.

Properly identifying the emotions to see if there are any themes, clusters or patterns will give you essential and valuable information for you to take and do something positive with. This may seem daunting, but keep with it as it will help you to clearly see what has been affecting you all these years so you can do something about it.

I created and devised this next exercise, Emotion Identification, to develop the Backward Step Technique exercise you have already done.

You may struggle with the exercises at first, most people do, because finally allowing yourself the space to focus on your psychological wellbeing is an unfamiliar and foreign concept to you. This is not self-introspection in a self-indulgent sense, it is about starting to focus on and consider all the things, big and small, that lead to your emotional eating, and finding your own personal way to overcome your destructive eating habits.

Emotion Identification

Step One

The Backward Step Technique exercise should have given you a clear idea of some of the emotional triggers of your eating habits. Look at the list of the actual emotions most commonly experienced and named by emotional eaters (see page 31) and think about what you felt last time you emotionally ate.

Step Two

Now, take out your notes from your Backward Step Technique exercise and pick out no more than three emotions that you most closely associate with each trigger/step you identified during the exercise. You may only associate one experienced emotion with what you have written on each step, or you may associate all three. You can repeat emotions for different steps too – in fact you are likely to have several repeating emotions. For example, you may have felt anxious in all steps, so it is okay to have the emotion more than once.

You may want to write down more than three experienced emotions. However, if you list too many you will be overwhelmed by them and you will end up with the 'What's the Point?' scenario where everything seems like too much to cope with. This is why you take this session in manageable and focused pieces, exactly as you would in traditional one-to-one therapy. It is important to focus on what you are hearing from a smaller group of identified emotions, so you do not feel overwhelmed. Emotion Identification is designed to be a very quick exercise where you are ideally aiming to name and identify the first instant and immediate emotions you think of in relation to the external trigger. Do not spend time pondering or correcting yourself; the aim is to get as accurate and realistic a list of the experienced emotions as possible.

Emotions Commonly Experienced and Named by Emotional Eaters

Abandoned

Alienated

Angry

Annoyed

Anxious

Belittled

Bored

Confused/Perplexed

Deceived

Defenceless

Deficient/Defective

Depressed

Despondent

Disappointed

Dismissed

Distressed

Embarrassed

Envious

Fearful

Flawed

Frustrated

Grieved

Guilty

Gullible

Helpless/Hopeless

Humiliated/Shame

Inadequate

Insecure

Insignificant

Jealous

Lonely/Ignored

Overwhelmed

Panicked

Pessimistic

Pointless

Powerless

Resentful

Resigned

Sad

Self-disgusted

Stupid/Foolish

Susceptible

Trapped

Uncertainty

Unimportant

Unwanted

Used

Voiceless

Weak/Fragile

Worthless/Useless

At first this exercise might be quite difficult to do, which is perfectly understandable, but do try to carry on. It is unnatural to want to revisit an emotionally painful time and recall everything associated with it, such as the negative feelings you had at the time, the eating and the shame of eating, which may themselves provoke new negative feelings. However, you will need to do this properly and accurately to identify what is really happening for you emotionally so you can start to do something about it. Let's return to our case studies, Kate, Frank and Linda, as they make links between their emotional triggers and their experienced emotions.

Case Study: Kate

'When I did the Backward Step Technique exercise, on my top step was the situation with the work colleague and her cake. The emotions that instantly spring to mind are **abandonment** and **rejection** because of how she treated me, and I felt **ignored** too, being left there all on my own. My second step was how I don't feel my husband always understands me that much. I feel I'm a bit **insignificant** to him, which then makes me feel **insecure** and **helpless** about my relationship with him. Next step was my belief that if my husband doesn't understand me, no one really can, and that makes me feel **insignificant** again and also quite **worthless** too. The fourth step of my list of contributing factors to my emotional eating was visiting my parents, which always makes me feel really **anxious** and **insecure**, but at the *same time rather **resigned** to it. Which brings me to the final thing on my steps list, my sister Emma. When I think about her attitude towards me it brings up so many emotions. For now, as I have to name just three, I would put **annoyed** and **defenceless** about the text she sent about me not doing enough for Mum and Dad's anniversary. Even though I have done lots she always manages to make me feel **guilty** as well.*

The reason why you are identifying your specific emotions is because they are part of the emotional chain of events. Doing the work to identify in detail the different stages of the emotional chain of events makes it much easier to take the opportunities at each stage to stop your emotional eating. If you can accurately identify your experienced emotions, you can then start to challenge, ignore or dismiss as irrelevant and untrue the message being sent from them to you. Just because these emotions are familiar it does not make them either true or the only type of emotions you are able to feel.

You are doing really well to be at this stage in the *Stop Overeating* plan, so start to introduce more positive emotions into your own internal dialogue – words and phrases such as being worthwhile, good enough or deserving are always a good place to start. There is still a lot of work for you to do, but it is never too early to feel positive and forward-looking, even if it is just a few internal phrases to begin with.

Case Study: Frank

'The first step on my list of triggering events is the relationship with my girlfriend and how it affects me. Firstly I feel very **inadequate** about it, **uncertain** and **fearful** about her, me and the whole relationship. My second step is not having many friends, which leaves me feeling **lonely** and **insecure** about everything, but **anxious** about being able to do anything about it. The third step is my lack of work and money, which leaves me feeling very **self-critical** that I should be doing more for my family, **inadequate** that I'm not a proper dad or partner. I'm really **fearful** of the future because I don't see anything really changing. The fourth step on the list is the supermarket petrol pump incident. Having to be helped by someone to get the cap off made me feel completely **useless**, **belittled** and just so **embarrassed**. I wanted to run and hide, which is what I did in a family-sized pack of tortilla chips two minutes later. My final step is my weight worries, which leave me feeling **humiliated** at being the weight I am, **helpless** as to what to do and very **anxious** about my health now and in the future.'

Some people experience distinct themes of emotions, others feel all sorts of different emotions – you do not necessarily have to be one or the other. However, if there are recurring themes in your emotional response, this is an indicator of where the issues are in your life that cause your emotional eating. Either way this exercise will be beneficial and useful because it gives you the chance to see where you need to focus your thoughts and attention towards stopping your emotional eating.

Case Study: Linda

'When I was told by the school about Jamie's poor work and bad attitude – my first step on the Backward Step Technique exercise – I felt really **distressed** and **fearful** about him and his future and also **guilty** that I have been letting him down, which is what I said to the teachers. Rob was the second step of the triggers of my food binges. He always makes me feel **worthless** because of the nasty things he says, then **stupid** because I always believe his excuses for treating me like he does, which then in turn makes me feel **trapped** because the only thing that ever seems to change in our relationship is my dress size. The third step was my work situation – this makes me feel **anxious** about not having enough of an income and **guilty** for not doing more to help my boss, but there is a bit of me that sometimes feels a bit **gullible** for being taken advantage of, working for nothing on occasion. My fourth step was having to look after my dad, which leaves me feeling **inadequate** and **self-critical** for not doing more, but at the same time he makes me feel really **belittled**, because he has always taken advantage of me, but then again that's my fault because I've never stopped him. Final step on my list was just never being in control of anything in my life, being useless at everything – my relationships with

> *Rob, Jamie and my weight. My eating makes me feel* **guilty**, **sad** *and* **anxious** *about everything going on and deep down I believe it's my own fault.'*

Like so many emotional eaters Linda has had such a lot to deal with throughout her life so it is hardly surprising she has such negative emotions about herself. Through no fault of her own, food has become her way of feeling and coping with what life presents her with. Linda does not have anyone but herself to rely on, and by being so negative about herself she could be in danger of taking away that option. However, she has taken the decision, no matter how long it takes, to identify and tackle the causes of her emotional eating, and by doing so she is strengthening her own self-resolve. Like Linda, being honest and reflective in what you feel emotionally is crucial in the whole principle and process of *Stop Overeating*, but just be mindful that you are not getting emotionally stuck there. Like Linda, Kate and Frank, you are learning to be not only your own therapist when emotionally provoking situations or encounters occur, but you are also becoming your own best advocate in these situations too.

You will look at the detail, the origin and meaning of these negative emotions and their subsequent messages in the next part of this session. For now, like Kate, Frank and Linda, you need to get used to naming and acknowledging the emotions themselves. Once you get into the habit of identifying emotions, you will be able to stop the emotional chain of events progressing any further so you do not get swept away by it and end up emotionally eating.

Part 3
The Negative Emotional Message and Your Relationships

In this final part of this Understanding the Emotional Chain of Events session you will look at two important aspects of your emotional eating that significantly contribute to it. Firstly, you will examine the real meaning of the negative emotional messages you receive, which is the last part of the emotional chain of events. These negative emotional messages are the result of the experienced emotions you identified in the previous part of this session. Secondly, you will start a detailed analysis and exploration of the relationships you have in your life to observe how they are a major influence on how you receive and accept the negative emotional messages in the first place. You will examine what has gone on for you in your relationships that makes it so easy for any negative emotional message to be received and believed, which of course in turn has the effect of continually undermining any long-term weight-loss efforts. You are using food to comfort yourself, to suppress the negative emotional messages you have received or as a form of punishment because you agree with what the negative message is saying about you – that you are defective, worthless and not good enough.

When you experience an emotion it will instantly send an emotional message to you about the original triggering situation or encounter. This emotional message helps you to make sense of what has happened or is happening to you. All emotions have a message attached to them, whether happy, sad, surprised, self-disgusted, guilty or anxious. For example, if you were walking down an unlit, lonely street after midnight (the triggering situation) and felt fearful (the experienced emotion) the message from the emotion of fear is that is it potentially unsafe and you need to quickly leave the street. It is exactly the same when it comes to your emotional eating: the emotional chain of events starts with a situation or encounter which triggers an emotional response, which in turn sends out a negative emotional message. But instead of a straightforward message telling you to leave the lonely and potentially dangerous unlit street, your emotional message becomes skewed, distorted and biased against you, becoming thoughts like *'You're defective for eating so much.'* Or *'You're not worthy enough to be slimmer.'* Or *'No one cares about you so why bother to do anything about your weight.'* These highly skewed and completely incorrect messages relay and mirror what are probably very familiar negative feelings you have about yourself. It is these types of negative emotional messages that constantly form, and add to, the idea you have of yourself and how you truly feel about yourself, which we call your self-concept.

Naming Your Emotions

I devised the Statement of Feelings exercise (see page 41), so you can examine the significance of your experienced emotions, and what it really means to you to feel and experience specific, or a group of, different emotions. Eventually you are going to be able to do your analyses really quickly, in just seconds, to stop any emotional eating.

For the Statement of Feelings exercise you will be working with the list of emotions you have named in the Emotion Identification exercise, so you can now start adding some meaning and significance to them. It is likely that at the time of the trigger event you had certain thoughts and feelings during or after it, but going back and making a detailed and comprehensive analysis of what the meanings may have been is a crucial part of stopping and managing your emotional eating altogether. Maybe, like Kate, you felt abandoned – her first identified emotion – because of a triggering situation, in her case the work colleague's cake incident. Kate also feels abandoned by her perceptions of her parents' attitude towards her. But what does feeling abandoned mean and say about herself to Kate? What is the actual meaning that is so intolerable that Kate has to eat to comfort herself because of it?

It's Not Going to Be the Same for All of Us

The meanings of your experienced emotions are going to be subjective, personal and unique to you. This is because being an emotional eater is a highly complex business – no two emotional triggers, let alone your response to them, are going to be the exactly the same.

Part of managing your emotional eating will be to see each emotional eating episode as unique. Do not be tempted to put them all together as you will be missing out on vital and important details, which you will need to know about to properly analyse the whole of your emotional eating. For now it is so important that you take the time to think through and honestly name the meanings and significance you attribute and attach to your experienced emotions.

Doing the Statement of Feelings exercise, like other exercises and features of *Stop Overeating*, will be psychologically uncomfortable. However, it is one of those 'darkest moment before the dawn' situations. You have to know what you are thinking so you can change and deal with it – something entirely within your power.

The negative emotional message is saying something distressing and very unwelcome both about you as a person and how you think you are negatively perceived by others close to you, a message that is usually highly inaccurate and does not reflect the real you at all. To overcome your negative self-perception you will need to do some honest thinking about the negative emotional message, what it is and crucially the origin of it, including who you believe has encouraged or dumped it on you. Without undertaking this level of honesty the danger is that the negative emotional messages will always have the ability to cause you distress and you will probably carry on having to eat to deal with them. Remember that, as you have already proved to yourself by getting this far in the *Stop Overeating* plan, you do have the psychological ability and strength to undertake and deal with your overeating, once and for all.

Statement of Feelings

Step One

Look back at the Emotion Identification exercise you completed, where you attributed your experienced emotions to the five external emotional triggering situations or encounters from the Backward Step Technique. Remember you are doing a whole chain of events analysis on one particular triggering situation or encounter so stay with the first one you have been working on. You will have come up with list of emotions from each step, so you have a list of emotions to analyse.

Step Two

For this Statement of Feelings exercise, you need to write three statements that best summarise what you are hearing from this list of emotions. You want an honest overall picture of how you felt about yourself at the time of the original emotional trigger. This could be something along the lines of: *'I'm not worth caring about'.* Or *'There is something wrong with me, I'm flawed and damaged in some way.'* Or *'It's my own fault, and I deserve everything I get.'* Or *'I don't have anything good or interesting to say.'*

These are the feelings and beliefs which are the cause of your emotional eating because it is these negative emotional messages that you cannot stand to hear, cannot cope with and cannot tolerate, so you eat to deal with them.

> ### *Case Study: Kate*
>
> *'When I look at my list of identified emotions (abandonment, rejection, ignored, insignificance, insecurity, helplessness, worthlessness, anxiety, resignation, annoyance, defencelessness and guilt) I hear a lot of negative messages from them. However, I need to look at them all together and come up with three sentences covering how they, and the original emotional triggering situations, make me feel. Firstly* **"I'm not worth caring about."** *Next* **"I'm invisible, not worth taking notice of."** *And finally,* **"There must be something wrong with me otherwise why would I feel like this?"** *This is how I've always felt about myself. It's a struggle for me to think about myself differently. I eat to try to make myself feel better but however much I eat, these feelings and thoughts never go away. Getting fatter gives me another negative emotion to feel about myself.'*

When you experience an emotional trigger that leads to an episode of overeating, with all its associated emotions, you get so caught up in what is going on that it is hard to think or feel logically or analytically about any of it, including the validity of your emotions or other people's agendas which may have been dumped on to you. Not surprisingly, afterwards you just want to forget all about it, but this will not help – you have to deal with all the causes of your emotional eating if you really want to stop it.

Only Three Statements?

It may be hard to think of just three statements about yourself which reflect the deep-down, long-held meanings of your experienced emotions. If you have too many Statements of Feelings, as with the other exercises you have completed so far, you will feel overwhelmed. The danger is that this could have a counter-effect and you may end up eating more to deal with it. Small and manageable steps forward will help you to stick to sustained long-term weight loss for the future. You will cover everything which is, and has been, distressing you at some point but it will be in a psychologically contained approach. Progressing slowly will allow you to build up a truly comprehensive picture of what has been causing and maintaining your emotional eating all these years. Think of it like learning to ride a bike or drive a car.

In her encounter with the work colleague and the cake, Kate quickly experienced the emotions of abandonment, rejection and feeling ignored. Even though the situation was not of Kate's making, as they often are not, Kate did not recognise the emotional trigger for what is was, namely the spiteful work colleague dumping her problems on Kate. Yet it is Kate who ends up experiencing the internal damaging emotions, which say something negative only about Kate, not her work colleague. This happens in all the steps in Kate's Backward Step Technique – the work colleague, her perception of her husband's attitude towards her and her parents' and sister's view of her. They all send loud and familiar negative messages to Kate about herself which she finds so upsetting that she emotionally eats to comfort herself from them.

Remember the emotional chain of events is just that: a chain, with one section linked to another. By analysing and identifying all the individual links, you can stop them connecting together and causing emotional eating.

Case Study: Frank

'When I did the Emotion Identification exercise I identified inadequacy, uncertainty, fear, insecurity, loneliness, self-criticism, uselessness, belittlement, embarrassment, humiliation, helplessness and anxiety. The negative messages I felt from them as a whole was that firstly, **"I believe I am damaged and flawed, that I'm no use to anyone."** Secondly, **"I can't provide for my family when they need me which makes me feel not good enough at all for anyone or anything."** And lastly, **"I feel like a complete coward, who cannot face any responsibilities and just goes to hide in a large bag of whatever is available or affordable."** These statements are nothing new; for as long as I can remember I've never felt good about myself, and because I don't feel good about myself how can I expect others to feel any differently about me?'

Being honest about what your negative emotions are saying is not going to be easy and will probably be psychologically painful too – useful and valuable therapy sometimes is. Maybe, like Frank, you have been avoiding identifying how you feel about yourself for many years, as a lot of we emotional eaters are prone to do. Remember, stick with it even if it is only a little bit at a time. As with lots of things which are worthwhile in the long run, this is going to be about both practice and exposure to distressing feelings, not doing what Frank has been doing all these years: suppressing and burying negative feelings with food. As you will know, it does not work – they are still there eroding your self-concept, your view of yourself, even after an emotional eating binge.

Case Study: Linda

'My main identified emotions from the Emotion Identification exercise were: distress, fear, guilt, worthlessness, stupidity, trapped, anxiety, gullibility, inadequacy, self-criticism, belittlement and sadness. I got lots of very familiar negative messages about myself from them – I've been used to feeling them for as long as I can recall. Sometimes these feelings may lose their intensity, but they're always there, lurking in my subconscious, infecting how I feel about myself. It took a lot to do this exercise, because being this honest about myself is not very nice, but I so want to do something about my emotional eating and weight. I know I have to. I've tried everything else over the years and it's not worked.

> *My first statement of how I feel from experiencing the emotions was:* **"Everything's my fault, I can't seem to do anything right, so it's not surprising others treat me like they do."** *Secondly,* **"I feel just so very weak and stupid all the time."** *And my final statement from my experienced emotions is simple,* **"I don't feel I really deserve anything better in my life. I should be fat and unhappy, because that's what I deserve."'**

The message Linda heard from her experienced emotions has been in place for many years due to her circumstances. If, like Linda, you find that you are making statements about being undeserving of happiness, remember that it is not you alone who is responsible for how you feel. Like Linda you may be trying to take on the responsibility for how others have acted towards you. In the final part of this session you will look at the relationships in your life to give you an insight as to how they can affect your emotional eating.

These are challenging exercises and you are doing really well to be undertaking them, so keep going because the information you are gaining is invaluable to managing and stopping your emotional eating.

If you do not feel quite ready to analyse your negative emotional message to this extent yet, that is okay. The negative emotional messages you receive and their meanings and significance to you have, after all, been a very powerful and destructive part of your psychological make-up for many years. It can be distressing to analyse them and bring them back to your consciousness when the emotional trigger situation or encounter and how you felt at the time has passed. So it is not surprising that all you want to do is forget about them, but, as your bathroom scales will tell you, this tactic of trying to forget about them has done little to help over the years. If you do not analyse or think about the negative emotional messages properly then the chances are that they will simply be allowed, albeit unconsciously, to keep influencing how you feel about yourself. In turn, this means that you will keep eating and using food to try to deal with your emotional response.

Stop Overeating is designed to offer you a level of emotional exploration as to why you emotionally eat in a contained and controlled way, not to provoke another emotional psychological episode. So remember to be kind to yourself, however unusual this idea of self-compassion is and however uncomfortable or self-indulgent it may feel to start with. Show yourself some long-awaited tolerance and consideration, and take things at a pace which is suitable for you.

Relationships

The damaging negative emotional messages that affect how you feel are biased against you. They only emphasise the negatives and ignore any positives. The messages are not usually at all accurate or truthful. So where does this psychological vulnerability to them come from? More often than not it will be your relationships which are a major cause. Your next step is to start analysing how the relationships in your life affect your emotional eating. How you feel about yourself, and how you feel others view you is an important continual cause of your emotional eating.

Your relationships, both past and present, are the foundation of what forms your self-concept. Remember your self-concept is both how you feel about yourself and how you believe others feel about you too. If it is at all distorted or damaged it will inevitably lead to vulnerability to any emotional problems, not just eating.

Any relationships you have are made up of two layers: firstly, your perception of your own particular place within that relationship, and, secondly, your perception, understanding and feelings as to how others in that relationship think about and view you.

Relationships of one kind or another – close, fleeting, distant, even past relationships – cover just about every aspect of everyone's lives. Even if you feel you do not have any relationships with anyone, or find it hard to sustain emotionally healthy relationships, that in itself will be because of how your previous relationships have affected you and made you feel both about yourself and others.

The Relationship Legacy

You will have various kinds of relationships which affect how you feel about yourself:

- **Work** relationships, such as with your colleagues, bosses, customers;

- **Romantic** relationships, such as with husbands, wives, partners, lovers, girlfriends, boyfriends;
- **Family** relationships, including with parents, siblings and your children;
- **Social** relationships, like with friends and acquaintances.

The relationships need not be lengthy: even people you sit next to on the bus or pass in the street have the potential to distress you in some way that ends up in emotional eating.

What you learn and accept from all of your relationships – close, distant, even brief passing ones – can be major contributing reasons for your emotional eating. Your relationships are at the foundation of how you feel about yourself. This is because how others treat you, whether it is fairly or unfairly, with respect for your abilities and intelligence or with no respect, with genuine interest in you or complete indifference, or with love, care and kindness or not, influence you. Your relationships are at the core of how you form a crucial inner understanding of yourself, your self-concept and the perceptions you hold about yourself. When your self-concept is a fragile one with a highly negative self-perception, this makes it much more likely that you will emotionally eat when it is damaged or threatened in some way by a triggering situation or encounter, which sets off the emotional chain of events.

From an early age all of us form an understanding and feelings about ourselves. This self-concept, the self-perception of how we feel about ourselves, including our strengths and our weaknesses, develops as we begin to test out our world and our place in it. Included in our self-concept are things like:

- *'Am I a worthwhile person?'*
- *'Do I deserve to be cared for?'*
- *'Am I important?'*
- *'Can I be loved by those who I believe should consider me important and lovable?'*

These all inform how you feel about yourself and what you feel is your place in the world. It is how you make sense of the world around you. So when the answer is 'no' to any of the above questions, or it is in doubt, this will of course have an impact on the forming of your self-esteem.

As you go through life you undergo a variety of experiences each and every day – at work, in school, with your relationships, family, friends and even people in the post office queue. In most cases a brief experience or interaction that you have is just that, brief and unremarkable, and is mostly quickly forgotten about or mentally filed away as inconsequential. The difficulty that emotional eaters have is they will take certain situations and encounters out of context, which adds to their low self-worth, their distorted belief that they are not worthwhile and do not deserve to be cared for. In its worst form, your damaged and fragile self-concept says *'I'm unlovable'*.

Case Study: Paul

'I never felt I matched up to my older brother's achievements, whether at school, at sport or at home. I was constantly compared to him, and as his little brother I was expected to be just like him. Stupid as it sounds this has coloured and affected my whole life. I became fat and overweight 40 years ago as a young child, because it was my thing, my individuality, the only thing that got me unique attention. It may have been critical attention, but it was attention nonetheless. My parents used to despair of me, and of course compared me to my brother, which was the worst thing they could do. I wanted them to know that, I didn't want to have to tell them. Everything just resulted in making me eat more. To this day, each Christmas they will still give me a low-calorie recipe book, a fitness DVD or gym membership. And any intentions I may have by myself, my own decision to do something about my weight are then buried in my renewed anger and resentment at them.

I feel like I'm having to reluctantly, and with enforced childishness, rebel against them all over again, to make myself be noticed for who I am, not what I am, which is an overweight, helpless 50 year old. I hardly have any contact with them throughout the rest of the year, but this brief contact at Christmas, or even the thought of it, makes me eat more just to prove the point that they can't influence me any more. But of course they do, because I'm emotionally eating each and every time I think about how my parents affect how I have

> *always thought about myself. It's definitely affected my*
> *relationships – I've never been able to have a successful*
> *relationship with any girlfriends, because deep down*
> *I don't believe they'd truly want to be with a damaged,*
> *fat, sad bloke like me when they could have a slim and*
> *successful bloke like my brother. It's how I've always*
> *seen myself.'*

Maybe you can relate to what Paul is saying. Even though his parents are in their seventies now, the relationship he has with them, albeit distant and fractured, still has a devastating and demoralising effect on him and how he feels about himself. Look at how much emotional control he feels he relinquishes to them, even if that is only once a year at Christmas. I particularly wanted to use the example of Paul because it shows that how you feel about yourself right from an early age can have a damaging effect throughout your entire life if you do not do something about it. Paul is in his fifties yet he feels like a worthless, useless child, who still compares himself with his older brother each and every time he has anything to do with his parents, which he subsequently emotionally eats to deal with.

Family Relationships

Although the effect and influence of all relationships are important, it is quite often your original family relationships which, like Paul's, are the most influential in your life, whether they were good, bad or you consider them indifferent. It will be your psychologically shaping family relationships, or in some cases the lack of them, which will have given you the original formative structure of your self-concept. Like it or not, family relationships, or the lack of them, are generally the template on which all other subsequent relationships are built. Negative family relationships have the potential to negatively influence a lot of your subsequent relationships.

It is widely accepted that children will form an inner concept of themselves during the first two or two-and-a-half years of life. This inner concept of the self will have its basis purely upon how others in their life treat them, particularly the principal caregiver, generally the mother. If the child has been treated with unconditional love, care and respect and their mother has been available to them, responding appropriately to their needs, then the child forms, a positive self-concept of themself and their environment. If the child has a stable and secure environment, they can then go on to explore their world in relative safety knowing they can always return to their mother if something goes wrong, or if something unexpected happens. The mother will give guidance, reassurance and boundaries so the child can learn from the unexpected experience and then carry on exploring their world securely.

This happens continually throughout life. If you are treated with love, interest and respect and are given genuine attention, as a rule you can generally form a rational understanding of the world and everything troubling or emotionally difficult which you come across throughout life. In other words you can usually cope with what happens to you without having to use food to comfort, suppress or punish yourself. You have learnt to build up some degree of resilience and have an aptitude to cope with potentially emotionally provoking events in your life.

If your personal experiences as a child, as a teenager or as an adult are those of insecurity, instability, conditional attention or unavailability towards you by significant people in your life, this will be damaging. It does not necessarily have to be highly abusive or neglectful, it can be far more subtle and less obvious, but it is your perception of those experiences which shapes how you feel about yourself, regardless of what others might or do say to counter it and subsequently make excuses for.

The Power of Relationships

Every time a situation occurs, or you have an encounter with someone which upsets or distresses you, the familiar negative emotional messages which underlie your poor self-concept are woken up, and the only way of dealing with the recurring negative messages they send to you about being useless, unvalued, not in control, not good enough, or unlovable, is to eat.

To illustrate how you absorb any negative emotional messages your internal emotions tell you about yourself, think about and remember yourself in the playground. Just about everyone who is an emotional eater has at least one painful playground experience to recall. Remember when someone, for whatever reason, called you something nasty, hit you or stole something from you, and remember how you felt when they did it to you. Perhaps you felt alone or stupid, sad or resigned at that time because of what was happening to you. It is the very same thing that happens each and every time your negative emotions are aroused or ignited by emotionally triggering situations. The negative emotional messages are just like the playground tormentor or bully. The negative emotional messages send a completely inaccurate message to you about being weak, stupid, unwanted, useless, but because of your influential formative experiences, which have shaped your negative feelings about yourself, you end up being very susceptible and sensitive to any damaging and harmful message your experienced emotions send. You believe them, you agree with them and you accept the negative emotional message about yourself.

As an emotional eater you continually do this because up until now you did not have the personal psychological resources, resilience or understanding of what was going on emotionally to be able to make sense of these inaccurate and harmful messages that your aroused emotions send to you. The only way you know to deal with them is in a temporary way by eating. Eating for comfort because of the harm the messages send, eating to try to suppress or divert yourself away from the messages, or eating because you believe the messages and feel you ought to be punished because of them. Of course whatever you do is only ever going to be a temporary fix, if it is a fix at all, because the underlying problems of how you feel about yourself remain.

The Relationship Analysis

Now you will start to examine, define and analyse your relationships to see how they are fuelling your negative self-concept and making it so easy for the inaccurate negative messages of your emotions to fit in and find a home. Quite often these are ongoing family relationships, and how you have been and continue to be perceived by others in your family is unlikely to change. But, and this is the crucial thing that will help you to manage being an emotional eater once and for all, how you perceive *yourself* in that particular relationship can most definitely change.

You do not have to be the person or fulfil the role subscribed to you by others. It can be your personal decision to change how you feel about certain situations or encounters. As much as the other people in your relationships may not like or welcome you changing, if you really want to stop your emotional eating you will have to make some attitude and psychological changes along with your actual diet changes too.

The Relationship Analysis exercise will take a straight-forward look at all the people in your life who you feel influence your self-concept and how you feel about yourself, as well as your subsequent emotional eating when you have had an encounter with them. This should include your family, work colleagues, friends or partner – anyone at all who has upset or distressed you to the point of emotional eating.

Relationship Analysis

Step One

For this exercise you will simply be categorising people in your life. You need to make two lists, firstly a list of those who are supportive, non-judgmental, genuine, caring and uncritical – the type of people who do not fuel, underlie or dominate your negative self-concept. The other category will be anyone, quite possibly close relatives and friends, who you believe, even if you have not acknowledged it before, you do not feel very comfortable with or around. The type who are uncaring or ambivalent towards you, untrustworthy, bullying, two-faced, judging and unsupportive of you.

Step Two

When you think about why certain people are on either list, where has your instinctive gut decision about them come from? What has your experience of them been in your life? The chances are that it will be borne out of your past experiences of them, like Paul, whose parental relationship was critical, judgmental and comparative to his older, successful brother. As Paul did when he was a child, and still does, he perceived it as conditional and rejecting. Because of these early relationship experiences, which have formed his self-concept and how he feels about how others would view him too, Paul has been unable to form many trusting adult relationships, as he feels he is or will be negatively judged and ultimately rejected all the time.

Step Three

On your lists look to see if there are any obvious and not-so-obvious connections between the unsupportive and untrustworthy people and the longer-term issues you have in your life, not just emotional eating. Do any of these people provoke something unwelcome and uncomfortable in you which perhaps has been going on unacknowledged for years?

Step Four

The Relationship Analysis exercise needs to be as automatic as possible. Try not to start making excuses for people's behaviour and attitudes towards and about you which have caused you to emotionally eat in the past. You are simply making a list of caring and not-so-caring, trustworthy and not-so-trustworthy, supportive and not-so-supportive people in your life. As you do it, look at the two different lists, think about the people on them. What makes them unsupportive and not so trustworthy?

Doing the Relationship Analysis and coming up with these two lists can often take a little bit of time, so do not try to rush it, as your categorisation of some of the people on your list may change. Someone who you may have thought of as honest and reliable to begin with is perhaps not so, and vice versa. As with every exercise in *Stop Overeating* it is really important to be honest about what you think. You do not have to show or discuss this list with anyone at all. You are compiling accurate lists of people who do, and do not, fuel your negative self-concept. These lists will help you to know who to approach or have around you when needed in the future.

Case Study: Kate

'When I did the Relationship Analysis exercise and made my two lists, I was surprised at quite how many people I would have just put down as okay for me to start with. But when I really thought about it they were not as entirely supportive as I feel they should have been. I had just assumed that because they were my family, they should be on the supportive list. For example my sister, Emma, who attention-seeks all the time, or my parents, who have always ended up giving her lots of attention to my cost. If I'm honest, usually when I have anything to do with my parents I do end up eating because they make me feel so insignificant and inferior. I don't think they mean to do this, but they do, as any conversation I can remember usually revolves around Emma – even from the first time I spoke about my wedding plans with them, they instantly wanted assurances that Emma was going to be chief bridesmaid and would have a major role to play in the whole wedding. On the supportive list, even though my husband doesn't always listen as much as I would like, he is very supportive of me and when I thought about it so are most of his family, especially and

> *somewhat ironically my new sister-in-law. It was a real eye opener to have her there genuinely supporting me in the run-up to the wedding. My new in-laws and friends seem to accept me no matter what, so it is good to know I have that proper understanding.'*

You are doing the Relationship Analysis exercise because if you can properly identify anyone who you feel is truly supportive of your needs and your efforts to lose weight then they are going to be a great source of support to rely on while you diet. It is a bonus to have external support, but not an absolute requirement. This is because you are much more self-reliant and capable than you have perhaps given yourself credit for over the years. Most people, even emotional eaters, are independent, self-sufficient and capable – it may have just been hidden for one reason or another for a long while so they never think of themselves in this way.

Case Study: Frank

> *'When I did my two lists I found it very surprising from both sides. My girlfriend, who, for all her problems, is supportive of me most of the time. My uncle, who owns an IT company and has got me a lot of work in the past, was someone I felt was a good support, which I'd never properly considered before. On the other list I put my mother, who is not really there for me when needed – she is always so wrapped up in her life. And she's always been funny about my girlfriend and children, making little*

digs and comments at them all the time. When I thought about my uncle being on the supportive list and my mum, his sister, being on the not-so-supportive, I was mentally able to divide them from each other, which I hadn't been able to do before. Even though Mum's a good 15 years older than him, in my mind up to that moment they came as one. Attributing them with opposite levels of support is a really useful thing to do. I know where to go for honest help and advice in the future when I need it, to my uncle, or girlfriend, not to my mother, who has very much got her own agenda for most things regardless of what that does to other people.'

If you can become aware of the past and present effects of some of your relationships on your emotional eating, you can do something about them. This does not have to be a dramatic cutting of all ties with people or sitting them down to tell them how you feel. It is more about an awareness of the potential that these relationships can have to cause emotional eating problems and therefore being able to equip yourself with the mental capacity to stop them by, if nothing else, just being ready for them.

Case Study: Linda

'I found this exercise really difficult to do, because even though they will never see it, or even know about it, I found it strangely disloyal to put some people on the non-supportive list, even though they deserved to go on it. After a bit of thinking I put my friend at work and

my boss on the supportive list, because when I have needed them in the past they have always been there for me. Over the years when I've needed to take time off because of Jamie being ill, my boss has been really good about it and my friend at work has covered for me, as I have for her when needed. Top of my non-supportive list was Rob. He really is not that nice to me, or supportive of me. I can't remember the last time he didn't make me feel bad about myself, let alone feel anything approaching good about myself, with his constant snipes and comments. Also on the unsupportive list are quite a lot of my family too, because, although I've had to be there for them plenty of times, my dad and my sisters either don't understand what it's been like for me all these years with Rob, and now Jamie, or they don't want to understand.'

Like a lot of people, Linda found this exercise hard to do, because she is a nice person and does not want to think badly of others. However, Linda worked through the exercise and came up with some interesting thoughts about who is and is not supportive of her. Ultimately, as is the case for all emotional eaters, Linda has herself to rely on and trust, which is something she has perhaps been overlooking. I designed this exercise to be practical, but also to be reflective. Like Linda you will need to properly reflect and understand that you are going to be your own best support and advocate. Having others is a bonus, but recognising your own self-supporting abilities is a vital part of overcoming your emotional eating.

If you find, like Kate, Frank and Linda, that you do not have too many truly supportive people in your life, it is not a problem. It simply emphasises that you need to rely on yourself in an emotionally triggering situation. They may not mean to, but others can let you down – it is highly unlikely that you will do that to yourself. For now, start to properly rely on and trust yourself. Remember it is you and you alone who will be eating and feeding yourself. It is great to have supportive people around you who value and love you, or even just take notice of you, but when it comes to the diet and weight loss, it is really only going to be down to you. You have to learn to be self-reliant, self-determining and independent of how others treat you. Understanding this is an important point as it will make you less reliant on and less fearful of others' opinions of you.

Often, finally getting to grips with and understanding the causes of and contributors to your emotional eating can be a psychologically changing experience. Just because you are making important discoveries and changes to your attitude and outlook does not mean that others will do the same; they will want to carry on as usual. You may be overweight and unhappy about it but this does not mean they have to change anything about themselves for you, even if they are a major cause of your unhappiness. Becoming aware of others' inflexibilities towards you will help you to stick with your diet efforts.

In this last part of Session One you have explored the final part of the emotional chain of events, the meaning of the negative emotional message. You have also begun to look back in your life at your relationships to see why the negative emotional messages always find such a willing home in your self-concept and how you feel about yourself.

You have already made massive progress in identifying the people and emotions that trigger your emotional eating. Learning about the personal reasons for your own emotional eating gives you the power to make changes for the future, and if you are following the 28-day Eating Plan you will be seeing physical as well as psychological changes. You should feel very proud of yourself for completing the first part of the *Stop Overeating* plan and taking the first major step towards a healthy and positive future.

session 2 / week 2
Me and Food, What Happened?

Introduction

In Session One, you examined how to identify the emotional chain of events, which included identifying the emotional trigger, the resulting feelings themselves and the negative emotional message you get from them. You have also started to explore the relationships in your life that have been a major contributor to your emotional eating. This week, you are going to be exploring how you have got used to using food to deal with your emotions in the first place. In this session you will look at some of the less obvious but very important factors that contribute to your emotional eating. Some may be more applicable than others, but this is your chance to explore some of the less straightforward and apparent causes and maintenance of your emotional eating.

You will explore the history of your poor relationship with food, where it has come from, who has encouraged it and why it has developed and remained such a problem in your life for such a long time. You will also look at how and why you have got used to using food to deal with your emotions, looking at particular habits, addictions and pre-occupations with food that are damaging to your weight. You already know that certain foods are fattening, are high in sugar and increase your weight, it is why and how you use food that needs exploring as well as some of the physically and neurologically addictive properties of the food itself. Finally, you will start to properly challenge your own beliefs about being an emotional eater. You will recognise and understand your entrenched and unhelpful beliefs about yourself and food so you can change them once and for all and stop emotionally eating.

As in traditional one-to-one therapy you will be building on the observations and discoveries you have made from the first session. This second session is again divided into three parts, which will make it easier to follow. You will continue to follow Kate, Frank and Linda to illustrate not only the exercises in each session, but also to give you a comprehensive understanding of what has made you an emotional eater.

Because you have got used to using food as a way of coping with upsetting and distressing things in your life, you never allow yourself the opportunity to deal with, tolerate and mentally process the uncomfortable emotional message you experience. By instantly trying to comfort yourself, suppress what you feel or punish yourself because of agreeing with what you feel, you never use any alternative ways of dealing with the distressing and upsetting emotional messages themselves, or their underlying causes. This is not unusual – if something or someone causes you pain, you want to eliminate, suppress or divert yourself away from the hurt as quickly as possible. So emotional eating has become your repeated way of dealing with the problems in your life. When you associate food, which for a brief moment or two is comforting or diverting and briefly conceals your emotional hurt and pain, that association becomes embedded in your subconscious. It literally becomes your default, and often only, way of dealing with emotional distress, upset and pain. No alternatives are considered or attempted. Add to that the enjoyable tastes of some foods, the pleasure some foods give, and it is a formula for a lifetime of weight issues and diet failures.

Part 1
Your Relationship with Food

In this first part of this session you are going to look at an important relationship you have as an emotional eater: your relationship with food. Your poor relationship with food is an established and constantly contributing reason for you being both an emotional eater and an unsuccessful serial dieter. Often emotional eaters will take the sole blame for how they behave with food, which is simply not true. As you have been finding out there are many reasons for your overeating and, like your relationships with other people, if you can evaluate your relationship with food and distance yourself from it when you need to, you will start to control it rather than let it control you.

Case Study: Miriam

'I've always had a love–hate relationship with food. I love certain foods, and when things get difficult at home – I'm a single mum with four teenage children – it's straight to the cheesecake. I can easily eat a whole one on my own in one go and it just takes away all the hassles for a short while. I know this attitude to food started when I was younger. My dad was an alcoholic and his behaviour was very unpredictable and volatile. I'd always be given money to go to the shop for sweets by mum, family and neighbours. They all knew how bad he was and I guess they felt sorry for me. And, yes,

> *eating used to help, still does to a point, but what it has done to my weight over the years is no help at all. So my relationship with food is conflicting: I hate food for what it's done to my weight, but I know I often rely on it for a few moments of relief from the never-ending chaos of my life.'*

Miriam is typical of a lot of emotional eaters. She has used food as a temporary solution and help with long-term problems in her life and historically always has done. However, as often happens for emotional eaters like Miriam, the food and eating has become a problem in itself. The weight, the self-criticism, the shame and regret are in themselves acting as an emotional trigger to the emotional chain of events, which Miriam ends up using food to cope with.

Like Miriam you will need to examine your relationship with food for what it is, which is likely to be a very well-established way of thinking with associated long-standing, but damaging, behaviours. Exploring your relationship with food will help you to reassess and change your way of thinking and behaving around food, which will ultimately play a part in helping you to lose weight once and for all.

Honestly examining your past relationship with food will help you in the future. In the first part of this week's session, you start by identifying any familiar themes and patterns from the history of your relationship with food so you no longer just have to follow familiar but damaging patterns unknowingly any more. Understanding your past food relationships and your conscious or unconscious attitudes which go with them are important because without proper examination they will continue to impact on your future relationship with food and eating.

Food Associations

The first exercise is called Real Food Relationships and helps you to discover what there is in your past relationship with food and eating that contributes towards you being an emotional eater, including your attitude and opinion of food and what you feel food and being an emotional eater have done to you in the past. This is so you can examine how your particular susceptibility to emotional eating has been formed, how and when you have used food emotionally and how this has then influenced your whole attitude to food and eating when something, or someone, upsets you. In other words, what does food and eating really represent for you? By examining your past, you will learn how to not instantly turn to food each and every time something emotionally distressing happens, just because that is what you have historically always done and, equally importantly, it has become what others in your life expect, and sometimes want, you to do as well.

Most people who have problems with their weight already know they overeat, but they fail to acknowledge both quite how far back their eating habits and poor relationship with food goes and quite how established it is. The more established and fixed it is, the harder to break. A lot of emotional eaters have unwittingly built up a lifetime's association with using and relying on food without even realising it. This poor food relationship greatly influences their emotional eating and is something which has remained un-investigated and unchanged, as has their weight problem.

Remember to take time to do the exercises in this session. Find somewhere that you will not be disturbed and can have proper thinking space. If you were having one-to-one therapy you would be getting your own dedicated time to consider what is and has been going on for you, so recreate it.

Your Food History

In this exercise, you will detail your past personal relation-ship with, attitude towards and use of food, making note of important times in your life when you recall using food to help you deal with problems. In the Real Food Relationships exercise you will assess how your food history began, what has shaped it and what has been added to it throughout your life. This will help you understand why you always turn to food when you have an emotionally provoking trigger event, so you can learn to make changes to your future relationship with it. Later on you will learn some psychological techniques and strategies to stop yourself from responding to 'in the moment' urges to eat. But what is important now is that you get a clear understanding of all the contributing aspects of your life, including your poor past relationship with food which underpins and facilitates your emotional eating in the first place.

Real Food Relationships

Step One

In this exercise you are going to be looking back to certain times in your life to examine how and why you have used food to help you. Think about your past in terms of:

a) Childhood

b) Teenage years/adolescence

c) Adult experiences with food and eating

Now, write down your thoughts about food during each of these times in your life, your associations with food and eating and what part it played in your life. Obviously there will be lots of memories and material for you to think about, however, try to be as succinct as possible.

Step Two

This exercise helps you to gain an overall view of what, and who, may have contributed to your own personal attitude and relationship with food, so you can modify and change it now and in the future. If names and places come up, make a note of them. If it helps, then use the 'five Ws' to prompt your thoughts – What, Where, When, Who and Why.

Let's return to our case studies of Kate, Frank and Linda as they undertake the Real Food Relationships exercise to see what findings they are able to take away.

Case Study: Kate

Childhood: 'I've always been quite shy and quiet, and if I had any difficulties at school, with friends, or at home when my older sister, Emma, was being particularly difficult, I learnt that a bag of crisps and a chocolate milkshake would make everything just a bit more tolerable. Mum would always have a plentiful supply for me because Emma, who was always so fussy about eating, seemed to hardly eat anything. I can remember from a very young age being encouraged to not be like her. Emma's eating, or lack of it, took a lot of attention from everyone, Mum, Dad, grandparents, teachers, so I took my attention and comfort from food. If I ate, Mum would be pleased with me, which would make me feel really happy.'

Teenager/adolescence: 'When I was at university, at least twice a week Mum would order my favourite pizza with all the extras, garlic bread, potato wedges, and have it sent to me in halls. I know I didn't have to eat it, but not only was it my favourite meal, but I felt I had to eat it as I'd be letting Mum down if I didn't. Emma was still at home then, still being really fussy over eating, and Mum would say she'd be happy if she knew at least one of her girls was eating properly.'

Adult: 'If I have any emotional, financial or practical problems at all I just instantly and automatically reach *for food to help. Even when I got married last year, all the associated stress that goes with planning a wedding was always dealt with by food. So much so, and to my disgrace and shame, that I had to get a bigger-sized wedding dress. The lady in the wedding shop even made a comment about it usually being the other way around – brides getting smaller dresses as the big day approached! I felt humiliated and angry at her for saying it, but more angry at myself for being so overweight. But, guess what, I ate again because of my anger. My husband always says he loves me no matter what size I am, and I know he's only trying to be supportive, but it doesn't always help much, especially when he gets me my favourite box of chocolates and bottle of wine to cheer me up.'*

Kate has been seeking comfort and relief in food since she was young, and like a lot of emotional eaters has a firmly established routine of repeatedly turning to food when she feels upset, ignored or humiliated, even at a really special time for her such as buying her wedding dress. Using food like this has been thought of by herself, and significant others in her life like her mother and husband, as her way of coping with problems. Kate has gone along with it because she does not want to make a fuss, but also because she does not know how and what to say to others to make them really understand how she feels. This only adds to the negative emotions she feels about herself.

Of course it is perfectly understandable that you have formed strong and abiding associations between food and emotions as we all have to eat from the moment we are born to survive. Like Kate, as a child you would have learnt to associate food with emotions of one sort or another, happy or sad, validated or ignored, loved or unloved. The problems often start in childhood when food is used by you, or others, as a form of control for your emotions. But it is when this bond with food, this really strong emotional association with it, becomes dysfunctional and is used for the wrong reasons that the damaging relationship begins and is maintained. It is natural to form some association with food for enjoyment, for pleasure or comfort, but it is when this association becomes the major reason for eating that your food intake increases because you need it more and more. This is where problems with your food relationship start, because you very quickly learn to use food as a substitute, a compensation for all sorts of deficits and problems in your life. Perhaps, like Kate, you comfort yourself by eating because of your vulnerability and your lack of confidence, which remains unnoticed by those who should be paying more attention to it.

Case Study: Frank

Childhood: 'My mum, who'd had me when she just turned 16, wasn't the world's best parent. She enjoyed her drink and boyfriends and quite often I would be in the house by myself, with a pile of toast in front of the telly and the dog for company. I'd often get left to it −

me, the dog and the toast — and when the dog died it was just me and the toast. I remember some teachers asking if I was alright, which although I wasn't I'd always say yes to, because I'd already had one horrible spell in a children's home when I was about six and I never wanted to go back there.'

Teenager/adolescence: *'As I got older it just continued. Mum was a bit more stable then, she wasn't drinking quite as much, and was always ready with a plate of chips, or bowl of ice-cream. If I had any difficulties at school or college that I found stressful, or if I ever tried to discuss her past behaviour and how it affected me, she would never talk about anything, brush it aside, laugh it off. Her favoured tactic would be to get the takeaway ordered and get the biscuits and crisps out while I waited for it to be delivered. She practically couldn't get the food in my mouth quickly enough to stop me asking awkward questions.'*

Adult: *'Now I'm an adult I can see where and why food and eating have played such an important role in my life. Food has been company and it's a useful device for not opening up to people — I learnt that very quickly from Mum. I do it to my girlfriend too. If she ever starts to question me about anything I find too difficult or uncomfortable, such as money, the twins or work, I will find something to cook, eat or go off to buy. I've learnt it's hard to really talk with something in your mouth. Food has been the one reliable constant in my life — it's always there, always available, it doesn't ask any questions or make any demands of me.'*

From an early age Frank was encouraged to use food as a substitute for what was missing in his life: the attention, interest and love from his mother. Food became a substitute for all that was lacking in his young, developing life. As he has grown older he has carried on using it as a substitute for lots of things. But for Frank food has also developed its own use as a diversion for when things get too uncomfortable, too difficult to discuss. Frank's relationship with food is one of reliance on it for so many things in his life.

Everyone has a history with food, even if it is one where you are genuinely not at all bothered about it. For emotional eaters that history will be complicated, in-depth and enmeshed with their emotional development from an early age. What has food and eating come to represent in your life? Attention? Comfort? A weapon to use to harm yourself and others with? Perhaps, like Frank, you have got used to viewing food and eating as a substitute for something missing in your life – an absent parent or a good job. Or maybe food has been encouraged by others to suppress your boredom, frustration, loneliness or lack of achievements.

Case Study: Linda

Childhood/teenager: *'If I look back I can see that food and eating has been an important tool for me over the years one way or another. My dad was verbally and emotionally nasty, always threatening to send me away somewhere if I didn't do what he wanted. I'm the last of three girls. Dad always wanted a boy right from the start, so when I came along as the last hope, he was really critical of me with hardly any interest or love at all. Mum died in a traffic accident when I was about seven, which left me really anxious at ever being left alone by anyone, ever. Although my older sisters did what they could, they both left home to get on with their own lives and in the end it was just me and Dad. Food was the one thing that made him human, especially his full English breakfast, which I became obsessed with making for him. If I did it right then he was nice; anything wrong and he'd be really horrible, calling me useless and stupid. Dad insisted that not only did I cook it for him each morning, but also that I sat down and ate it with him too – he never liked to eat alone. If the breakfast was okay and he was being nice, I was all too willing to be there eating as much as I could, keeping him nice for as long as possible. Thinking about what to do for dinner or breakfast each day became my daily task, because as long as the meal was nice, then there was the possibility that Dad would be too.'*

Adult: *'When I met my partner, Rob, not surprisingly I jumped a bit too quickly at the chance of getting away from Dad. For a while it was fine, and without really trying I even lost quite a bit of weight when we were first together. But when Jamie was born Rob became just as nasty and vicious as my dad, ironically saying that he had really wanted a girl, as he's already had two boys from a previous relationship. He started saying* *how useless I was, what a rubbish mother I was and was always threatening to find a better partner for himself and mother for Jamie. I'm not sure quite what I do that's wrong, but again and again I just manage to bring out the bad in everyone, even my own son. He's always making horrid comments about my weight, saying how badly I compare to his friends' mums. But then behind his back I go and get as much food as I can eat to deal with what is going on in my heart and my head. I always have, it's the only way I know to deal with the difficult things in my life. I never really enjoy the food I binge on — I wouldn't want to enjoy it, I don't deserve it.'*

From a very early age Linda suffered psychological abuse and neglect and formed a deep-rooted association with food as a temporary escape from her father's nasty attitude towards her. As food helped with her anxieties about being left alone without her son and her partner's constant threats to find someone better, it is imperative that she understands that she has the psychological ability and resources to overcome and learn how to manage her anxieties in a way which does not always have to involve food.

When others in her life, her dad, her husband and son call her names, abuse her, belittle her because (through no fault of her own) Linda does not know any differently, she unhappily goes along with their view of her, as someone who deserves to be criticised and bullied because of her many perceived flaws. However, Linda also uses food because she is fearful of being left on her own, wrongly believing it is better to have someone around, even if they are belittling, than no one.

Your past and present relationship with food will be as in-depth and complicated as all the other relationships you have in your life. It will probably have firmly established themes and patterns, you will have got used to using food to solve or help with many different types of problems and issues in your life. But all too often and all too quickly, the very thing which briefly helps to deal with a problem, to cope with an issue, soon becomes the problem itself. Food has become its very own external emotional trigger, the shame attached to it, the anxiety of being caught eating, the depression at being overweight, so that emotional chain of events never seems to end. By looking at and uncovering your history with food and your attitude towards it you will really be able to do something about it – change your attitude towards food and change your relationship with food, which will all go towards helping you to stop gaining weight and become a successful dieter.

Obviously you are still going to have to eat, you cannot simply abstain, or give up eating like you can with smoking and drinking alcohol. Becoming conscious of the dangers of what has gone on in your past relationship with food, so it no longer happens in the future will be a fundamental help to stopping emotional eating. Examining where, why and how long this poor relationship with food has been around in your life will ultimately help you do something challenging and positive about it. If you can truly see it for what it is, you will understand, have some self-compassion and stop being hard on yourself, because of how difficult you find it to lose weight and maintain your diet. Remember, most people will diet at some point in their lives and it is a challenge for everyone, not just emotional eaters.

Undertaking the *Stop Overeating* plan is hard work, so remember to make sure you give yourself some acknowledgement of your effort and dedication, even if it just a metaphorical pat on the back. It does not have to take any more than a few moments to tell yourself how well you are doing. It would be great if others did too, but being able to encourage and affirm yourself is going to be really beneficial both psychologically, with the *Stop Overeating* plan, and physically too if you are following the 28-day Eating Plan.

Part 2
Habits, Addictions and Pre-occupations with Food

In this part of Session Two, you will explore your habits, addictions and pre-occupations with food and see how one or all of them have affected your eating and weight problems. There are no exercises to do in this part of the session because, as in traditional one-to-one therapy, it is helpful to have some purposeful time to reflect on your progress with the plan so far. You have been working really hard, completing very emotionally challenging exercises, working through lots of sensitive and detailed information and crucial psychological insights to the reasons why you have become an emotional eater.

Observing and exploring habits, addictions and pre-occupations with food will give you the opportunity to gain important and valuable knowledge and awareness of all the potential but often unacknowledged contributors to your emotional eating. This will help you understand why you think, act and behave in such a damaging way with and around food. Some of these topics may not be relevant to you but it's important that you view this part of this session as a really valuable time to think about both what you have already achieved and the next part of stopping emotional eating. It is important not to lose the continuity of your sessions, but equally it is important to review and reflect on what you have found out so far.

Habits

Emotional eaters often have many eating habits, from always turning to food when they undergo an emotional provoking encounter, to constant eating and grazing which has become automatic. It is hardly surprising that so many people find it hard to break dysfunctional and damaging eating habits with food, as there is always so much of it about. If it is not physically in front of us, then food is being advertised or promoted to us all the time in other ways. In today's world we have all become used to, and conditioned into, rarely going more than a few hours during waking hours without eating or having something in our mouths – at home on the sofa, in front of the television, at work at our desks, during social events or at the cinema, where some food is available in buckets. But for those of us who have problems with weight loss and dieting, not only are these constant opportunities damaging to our weight but there are very few things we are going to eat on these occasions that are not fattening and weight-increasing to some degree or another.

For emotional eaters having this plentiful and available supply of food is really difficult because when you have a situation or encounter set off your emotional chain of events, it is just too hard not to indulge in what is so readily available. Even if it is high-calorie, high-fat and low-nutrition food, which you know is damaging. After what is probably a lifetime's habit of turning to this type of food when you get upset or distressed, these are the habits which are going to be hard to break, but with the right monitoring and management they are breakable and controllable. Assimilating the information from your discoveries so you can incorporate new thoughts, behaviours and attitudes to both your relationships with others and your relationship with food, you will be in the very best place to overcome your past eating habits and undertake a weight-reducing diet successfully.

Case Study: Kate (Habits)

'As soon as anything happens to me that I find distressing, upsetting or even just slightly uncomfortable I know I grab the first thing I can get hold of to eat. And I know I do it if there is also something coming up, like the visit to my parents for their 30th anniversary that I'm anxious about. The thought of having to deal with my older sister, who still lives at home, has me practically running to the fridge on an hourly basis. It was ironic that when the work colleague came in with the cake and didn't give me any, all I wanted to do was run over to it and grab the biggest slice I could, firstly because of the upset of the situation and wanting it to comfort myself, but if I'm honest because it's what I always do: eat. I spend hours of my day either eating something fattening or drinking endless coffees and hot chocolates at work and then wine in the evening. Plus, of course, every glass of wine has to be accompanied by a bowl of crisps, nuts or olives. It's become such a habit it would feel odd not to be eating or drinking something all the time. I've always thought

*it was just my emotions that have been the cause of
my overeating, but if I'm honest I eat all the time out
of habit anyway, it's just that I eat a lot more when I'm
emotionally upset.'*

When you think about habits, it is not just about the physical habit of eating. Perhaps like Kate you have also got into the habit of using food before any situation or encounter has actually happened. Kate has quite a few ongoing situations in her life which she finds difficult to tolerate or think about objectively, so she is in the habit of eating before any emotional situation has arisen. Just the threat of them is enough to get her emotionally eating. Of course, on the occasions when the anticipated event does not happen or it is less emotionally provoking than she had thought it was going to be, Kate potentially ends up in the position of then being self-critical and giving herself a hard time for having eaten unnecessarily in the first place, which of course is potentially another trigger for the emotional chain of events.

Think about the last few days and how long you normally go between either eating or drinking something. More than likely it is not going to be that many hours, apart from sleeping. This is the type of habit you will need to properly identify so you can break it and lose weight. You will have to stop grazing and mindlessly eating unnecessary food, which may be a challenge. Even if you are not eating for emotional reasons, it is hard enough to stop, but throw in some emotionally provoking situations or encounters and it is going to be made all the more difficult. But now that you are learning the tools to identify emotionally provoking situations and encounters you are starting to understand how to manage them more successfully.

Addictions

Addiction is an emotive and forceful term with many negative connotations. A lot of people only associate addictions with substances like drugs or alcohol, but there is plenty of scientific research that suggests physical food addictions are just as strong. The intense motivational need to seek certain foods is just as strong as it would be with cigarettes, alcohol or drugs. This is why sometimes you feel that certain foods are literally talking to you, requesting to be eaten, and you feel powerless to resist.

Viewing food as an addiction can give you some interesting, helpful and useful knowledge about what your motivations really are. It is not just your emotions on their own which cause overeating, and there can be other exceptionally strong physical motivators that are significantly influential as well. When in the past, as you have undoubtedly done, you have tried to abstain from certain foods, you have probably found it virtually and ridiculously impossible to do. Having this knowledge of why it is so hard, especially when you are emotionally vulnerable, should help you to stop feeling like there is something wrong with you.

Case Study: Frank (Addictions)

'I hate it when I drive past a certain fast food shop near where I live, because it's almost like I become possessed by the thought of it. Up until that point (if nothing too stressful has happened) then I'm not really thinking about food or eating. The moment I see the familiar bright boarding it just seems to set something off in me. No matter how hard I try to fight it, I have to have some and sure enough I'm in the queue for the drive-through before I know it. It's not just fast food I crave, although I think that is a major cause of my massive weight problems, it's anything at all I know I get some satisfaction from. The moment I see anything associated with a certain food, even a brand colour for certain chocolates, I just have to have some of it.'

Frank does have choices: he does not have to eat all the food which is so harmful to his weight, his health and his psychological wellbeing. However, after a lifetime's exposure to such addictive foods it is not going to be easy for him. He will need to be very aware, not only of what is going on emotionally, but what is going on physically and neurologically, as well. He will need to make sure he always has sensible amounts of healthy foods to hand as an alternative to satisfy his cravings. If he does not, his addiction to certain foods will keep harming his weight-loss plans and it will be a lot harder to lose and maintain any weight loss in the long run.

Pre-occupations

You can form pre-occupations with food and eating for a number of reasons. Maybe it is because of pleasant, enjoyable or emotionally relieving associations with a past experience, which you are trying to repeat. Maybe it was a happy time, or maybe it was a time when emotionally eating worked for a little while, when it helped to temporarily deal with the negative emotional message you received at the end of the emotional chain of events. People who develop a pre-occupation with food are continually striving to recreate one or more previous experiences, where they believed food and eating benefitted them in some way.

Earlier, Linda mentioned how the only time her dad was nice, and not hostile towards her, was when she had cooked his breakfast for him in an acceptable way. By obsessing and becoming pre-occupied by food she is trying to recreate that sense of reduced anxiety and satisfaction she felt then when she eats now. Since eating was the only time she was not being verbally abused, Linda is continually chasing those elusive moments of relief with food.

Case Study: Linda (Pre-occupations)

'The only time my dad was ever okay with me, didn't berate me or call me stupid, was when I made his meals. If I got anything wrong with his full English breakfast, the eggs too hard or the fried bread too soft, it would get thrown straight in the bin and he'd just revert back to his horrible self. And it was the same with my partner, keeping him well fed kept him reasonably happy,

especially when we first got together. So from an early age I know I've always been a bit obsessed with keeping everyone happy with food, because if they were happy then they were not being quite so horrible. If things go wrong with anything in my life now it's my automatic reaction to find food and stuff myself silly. And if I don't have anything in, I'll be thinking about it. I've often gone to a 24-hour supermarket to stock up on cakes, crisps, sausage rolls and chocolates. When I say "stock up" I mean eat most of them on the way home. On one hand I'm trying to make myself feel better with food, but deep down I know I don't deserve to feel any better because I get so much wrong, so much of the time. Getting fat is the price of that.'

Having a chance to think about what is happening habitually (behaviourally), addictively (neurologically) and with any pre-occupations you have about food (mentally) will give you crucial knowledge and information to be able to stop it. Any habits, addictions and pre-occupations will only become worse and affect your nutritional eating, as well as your emotional eating, unless you take the time to identify and do something about them before they take over all of your eating and negatively influence your relationship with food for good.

Examining these habits, addictions or pre-occupations with food is your chance to think about, and reflect on, what food and eating has meant in your life so far, which is very much a part of any traditional one-to-one therapy. Maybe you habitually eat when you do not need food for nutrition, or you have developed an addiction to certain foods without really knowing or understanding it. You are certainly not alone if you have. Or perhaps your pre-occupation with food has become the dysfunctional all-consuming focus of your relationship with it. Some of these may not be applicable to you, but *Stop Overeating* is about making sure you cover all bases concerning the potential contributing causes of your emotional eating.

Knowledge is power as they say, and having knowledge about any potential contributory factors to your emotional eating will be your power and your control to become a successful dieter with long-term sustained weight loss.

Part 3
The Beliefs of an Emotional Eater

So far in this session you have already examined your poor and damaging relationship with food, your habits around and relating to food, the neurologically addictive properties of certain foods and how, as an emotional eater, you can develop unhealthy and unwanted pre-occupations with food and eating because of its associations with past emotional experiences. Together, and separately, all of these play a role in your emotional eating. However, other strong contributors are the firmly held beliefs you will have about being an emotional eater in the first place, including how it may benefit you as well as cause you the problems it does.

When I first see people for therapy for overeating, a lot of people do not say they are seeking therapy for their weight issues initially, which is understandable because of the shame involved in being a compulsive overeater. As an overeater the sense of shame covers so many different things: a level of self-hatred for allowing yourself to get in this situation in the first place, regret of being like it, loss of control and the loss of what you could have been. And any sense of shame is perpetually compounded by your inner critical voice. However, what I always tell my clients when they talk about the sense of shame they feel, is that it is never just them alone who is responsible for how they feel at that particular time. Granted, it is them who have put the food into their mouths, but there is just so much more underlying that action, it is disproportionate and wrong to lay all the responsibility on their own shoulders.

Quite often people will say they are seeking help for depression or an anxiety problem of one kind or another, and if that is what they want to work on at that particular time then that is where we leave it. And of course depression and anxiety are often wrapped up with weight problems and subsequent emotional eating and may need addressing as concurrent or separate issues. However, because these types of psychological presentations are not exclusive to weight issues, it is often useful to try to separate them to work on therapeutically if the client wants to. Obviously certain psychological issues in your life are linked to others, which then in turn all impact on further troubling issues, but unless you start by focusing your attention on different problems separately as much as possible, especially at the beginning, you will find it really difficult to progress on any issues that are causing you problems in your life apart from emotional eating.

When I see someone for therapy for emotional eating, whether or not they say it is weight-related to begin with, I will ask what they feel are the reasons for their psychological problems. Generally, with people who have sought help for their weight, soon after we start therapy the topics of weight and emotional eating are discussed. Over the years I have heard many wide and varied explanations as to what people believe is the reason for their emotional eating. I have heard people say they believe their overeating is caused and maintained individually or as a combination of social problems, financial issues, or just the convenience and abundance of fattening foods available.

All of these reasons and explanations are valid and true to some degree, some people do even acknowledge psychological beliefs they hold about being an emotional eater when they begin therapy, however this psychological understanding tends to be fairly limited or too focused on one particular cause, such as not having a job, their partner leaving them or stress caused by children. Believing that your emotional eating is caused by one or two specific reasons will allow other unacknowledged causes and contributors to your emotional eating to increase and continue, unrecognised and unchallenged, to influence your damaging emotional eating. By now you should be getting used to properly identifying causes and emotionally provoking triggers for the Backward Step Technique exercise you did at the beginning of the Understanding the Emotional Chain of Events session.

The Truth About Your Beliefs

Contrary to what either others may have told you or what you may believe yourself, simply eating too much and doing too little exercise, having no self-control or willpower is not the classic recipe for being overweight and useless at diets. There is nothing simple about being an emotional eater. If it was simple then you, me and every other emotional eater would have done something about it years ago and you would not be in your current predicament seeking professional help for it. Emotional eating is psychologically very complex; it is a state of mind where everything emotional seems to get mixed up and confused along the way, but it always results in the same thing: you being overweight and unhappy about it.

In this section you will carry on unravelling and identifying any causes of your emotional eating. Specifically you are going to tackle some of the beliefs you truly hold about yourself, and, importantly, some of the beliefs you believe others hold about you and your emotional eating. This will help you gain an understanding of how these beliefs are another contributor which is continually adding to, and helping to cause, your emotional eating.

Following the examples of Kate, Frank and Linda you will explore the three most often reported areas of beliefs about being an emotional eater:

1. Your Identity as an Emotional Eater

Do you feel as if, over the years, the real you has somehow got lost in the emotional eating you? Perhaps you have lost sight of who you are and what you have become, namely an emotional eater.

2. Secondary Gain

As an emotional eater you may gain certain benefits. As well as consuming food that you like the taste of, you may also gain other benefits like not working, not forming successful romantic relationships or friendships, being looked after by others or being left alone.

3. Fear and Concerns About Trying to Stop Emotionally Eating

Here you will take into consideration your relationship with food and any past failures and disappointments with your diets and weight-loss attempts which add to your fears.

Beliefs

Step One

For this very simple and straightforward exercise, all you need to do is think honestly about all the beliefs and feelings you have about food as well as your beliefs about being an emotional eater. Remember this is for your eyes and thoughts only, no one is going to see them, judge them or comment on them so be honest with yourself. Maybe you believe that emotional eating and the anxieties that surround it stop you from having to socialise, or your emotional eating means you do not have to be with someone who you do not want to be with. Or perhaps you believe that trying to stop emotional eating will then deny you your favourite foods and tastes, which deep down you do not want to give up.

Step Two

Now write down your beliefs somewhere private. Remember that this is about identifying and being honest about the hidden reasons why emotional eating is controlling you. Use the headings 'My Identity', 'Secondary Gain' and 'Fears and Concerns about Trying to Stop' to help. If you are struggling, write down a few sentences that begin *'My honest and truthful belief about me being an emotional eater is ...'* and fill in the blanks under each heading.

As with all the other exercises in *Stop Overeating* there is no right or wrong answer, this is simply about gaining as much open and truthful information as you can about the different contributors to your emotional eating and weight problems. That is the rationale for this exercise – to be fully and honestly aware of your beliefs, both so you can start to challenge them and also to be aware of them so any unrecognised harm they have been doing ceases.

Case Study: Kate (Identity)

'When I did the Beliefs exercise a few things came up about what I believe and feel about food. Firstly that when I'm anxious, scared of something or someone, I believe that food is my one and only option, it is reliable and, unlike some of the people in my life, is always available to me when I need it. The other main finding was the fact that I believe I'm someone who can't cope without food. It's become very much part of who I am to myself and I guess to others. It's become my habit to turn to food all the time when something upsets me.

So it's hardly surprising, although saddening, that others in my life, including my family and my husband believe this about me. They all seem to think if I'm having a problematic time, pass me a large bar of chocolate and a bottle of wine and I'll be fine, which of course I never am, just a bit fatter and a lot sadder.'

Kate believes that many people, including herself to some degree, believe she is unable to cope with emotionally provoking events without always turning to food. It has made it hard and difficult for her to stick to and succeed on a weight-loss plan. Kate believes that being like this is part of who she is, however coming to an acknowledgement and understanding of this belief will help her to start to challenge it. At the moment it may only be Kate who challenges these beliefs, but by doing so she will be greatly helping herself to lose weight without the added difficulty of fighting an inaccurate belief of herself as a person who cannot manage without food.

Case Study: Frank (Secondary Gain)

'My main belief about being an emotional eater is, if I'm really honest, that it has stopped me from having to achieve anything with my life. If I've got my head stuck in a burger and fries then I don't have to think about anything else, like a decent career or being a proper provider for my girlfriend and children. I've never been that social or comfortable around new people, and when I've tried to get various jobs over the years or go to

college, I've found it stressful being around strangers. I usually end up coming home via the chip shop and give up altogether. Mum used to say that I didn't have to try again, it was okay to be at home with her. Looking back I can see this didn't do me any favours, then or now. When I did move in with my girlfriend, Mum wasn't best pleased.'

Your emotional eating, and perhaps the subsequent weight gain, could be acting as your armour, your defence against situations or encounters you do not want to have, or be involved in. Frank eats because he feels stressed and anxious in certain social situations, but he also benefitted from eating: he no longer had to face these high-anxiety provoking situations. Also he calms his anxiety by eating the type of food he enjoys and wants. These are some of Frank's secondary gains of being an emotional eater. Perhaps you can relate to his example? Being an emotional eater can be beneficial because it stops you doing something which you do not want to do, like going to college or getting a job in Frank's case. Admitting that you eat to seek the benefits of avoiding and doing certain things in your life, or to gain attention and concern, can feel strange. Harming and sabotaging your own health and wellbeing by overeating is not something many people want to admit to themselves, let alone others. Yet it is one of the important factors of emotional eating and you will go on to cover the whole aspect of self-sabotage in the final session in more detail. For now having honest thoughts about any secondary gain you get from being an emotional eater will be very important to taking control of your eating habits.

> ### Case Study: Linda (Fear and Concerns)
>
> *'I don't believe that I use food for comfort, in fact it's the opposite. When something bad happens to me I believe I overeat food to confirm the feelings I have about myself, that I'm totally rubbish and completely stupid. I believe I'm a damaged person – ever since I was born I've been getting things wrong. Dad never stops reminding me, even now, that I should have been a boy and what a disappointment I was right from the start. I believe I deserve to be exactly what I am, fat and unhappy. And I know that if I did try to do something about my weight I'd only fail again, and that's too scary to even think about, yet another failure in my life.'*

As Linda's comment shows, being an emotional eater is a very complicated way of living; it impacts and influences so many things in your life, not just how and what you eat. Like Linda, many emotional eaters hold the belief that their situation is solely their responsibility. It has become their default way of thinking, which in itself is not their fault. Linda compounds her thoughts about herself by referencing situations and events from long ago, such as her father's attitude towards her from birth. This is common with many emotional eaters because in a way it helps them cope, it is that little bit of control, the 'jump before being pushed' way of thinking. Because if you can think and say all the horrid things and thoughts to yourself first, psychologically it just makes it that little bit less devastating when someone else does. Especially if they are supposed to be someone who should have your best interests at heart, such as Linda's father.

Emotional eating has been a constant, albeit an unwelcome one, in your life for many years, and perhaps even the thought of failing at doing something about it is full of fear. Fear, of course, is a powerful emotion in itself, which could easily set off the whole emotional chain of events again, ending in another unwelcome and distressing negative emotional message being sent about you. So it is of little surprise that people who have such rigid beliefs and negative internalised views about themselves, and their likelihood of failure, do not want to even try anything which may be good and useful to them, such as dieting and losing weight.

Believe in Yourself, You Can Do It

The one thing that can alleviate your fears of failure about stopping your emotional eating and losing weight is a new, positively modified belief in yourself, which you are learning throughout this book. Remember, if you do not try to do something about your fear of failure nothing will change for you, your beliefs about being an emotional eater or your weight.

Undertaking the Beliefs exercise is about seeing whether the beliefs you hold about being an emotional eater are true and whether they still serve the purpose you believed they once did. Maybe you are like Kate, and being an emotional eater gives you an identity where you, and others in your life, believe that you cannot cope without certain foods. Perhaps you can identify with Frank, who has a secondary gain from his emotional eating. He believes that because he is overweight and because of his emotional eating, he is stopped from doing and achieving certain things in his life that he would otherwise do. Or you may be like Linda, where your fear of failure is so strong and overriding that you fear doing anything about your emotional eating in the first place, because failing at it is too much to contemplate.

To finish this session, ask yourself about the benefits and costs that your beliefs about yourself cause. Be honest and see if anything new comes to light.

This session has explored and examined some of the not-so-obvious aspects of being an emotional eater, which all contribute to your emotional eating and weight gain in the end. Remember, *Stop Overeating* is trying to cover every aspect and contributory feature and factor of being an emotional eater. Some may not apply to you, or all of them may be applicable. However, it is important to consider them all, because there could be something which you have yet to fully acknowledge. The unacknowledged causes and contributors to your emotional eating can be the most dangerous because if they remain unexplored they have opportunity to carry on unchallenged and unchanged and you will find sticking to a diet and losing weight so much more difficult.

Well done, you have now completed Session Two, and are halfway through the plan. Keep going, because between the *Stop Overeating* exercises, the 28-day Eating Plan and, most importantly, your hard work, you will be feeling the benefits of what you have done so far.

session 3 / week 3
Start to Stop

Introduction

In Session One, you uncovered and explored the three psychological components of the emotional chain of events that has resulted in your emotional eating. Then in Session Two, you honestly explored your relationship with food, any contributions from habits, food addictions and pre-occupations to your emotional eating and what your own beliefs are about being an emotional eater. In this session, Start to Stop, you will be learning short- and long-term strategies to curb and stop your emotional eating.

When you experience an emotional chain of events, you need to know what to do about your emotional eating urges in the short term, the actual there-and-then moment, to stop you turning to turn to food and eating to deal with the damaging emotional message you are receiving from your felt emotions. The first exercise in this session – called the Mini Moment Intervention – will teach you how to stop and control the urge to emotionally eat when a situation happens. The second exercise – called the Maxi Effect Analysis – is where you will begin to examine the long-term contributors to your emotional eating in detail, so you can at last be in a position to challenge them.

The Mini Moment Intervention is like having a brief call to your therapist to stop the urge to emotionally eat, and the Maxi Effect Analysis is like having a full one-to-one session with your therapist.

In the final part of this session you will learn how to begin to effectually and accurately challenge any negative emotional messages you receive, which, remember, is the net result of the emotional chain of events. Analysing and challenging the harmful messages is a crucial part of stopping your emotional eating once and for all.

Part 1
The Mini Moment Intervention

You are an emotional eater because up until now, through no fault of your own, you have lacked the ability to tolerate, process and challenge the negative emotional messages that certain situations or encounters bring up for you. The urge to emotionally eat is usually fast, unconscious, repetitive and automatic. This can be a here-and-now urge: the type of feeling which you try to deal with using food at the moment of, or very soon after, the external emotional trigger has set off the emotional chain of events. Or you may be a planner, the type of emotional eater who stores up the negative emotional messages, spending time ruminating and thinking about everything in the chain of events and planning your emotional eating for a time not too far in the future.

Planning to Emotionally Eat

Planning to emotionally eat like this is more frequent in, but by no means exclusive to, those who use food and eating to punish themselves, because they fundamentally agree with the negative emotional messages received. Through planning the damage and harm you are doing to yourself by emotionally eating, blowing the diet and gaining weight, you are then not only adding to your fragile self-concept and low self-esteem, you are also agreeing with the original negative message about yourself. It's just another one of those vicious circles that emotional eaters have to endure on a regular basis.

> ## Case Study: Graham
>
> *'Recently a friend who I'm very close to asked if he could stay over for a week while he had some building work done. I spent ages cleaning and tidying up, making the spare room nice – no mean feat when it's been a dumping ground for years. I don't usually bother with breakfast, but I got his favourite breakfast cereals in as well. At the last minute I got a text to say he'd had a change of plan and was going to stay with his parents instead as he didn't want to put me out. It made me feel so unimportant and disposable. For the rest of that day I thought about nothing else but going to the supermarket and getting more boxes of the most calorific cereal I could find and lots of full-fat milk and sugar. And then I spent the entire night alone in my kitchen eating all the cereal I'd got in for him, as well as all of the ones I'd got on my way home from work. I spent hours eating it all and only stopped when I felt I was going to be sick. I felt so taken for granted, so undermined and useless.'*

Graham is typical of someone who plans his emotional eating. He experiences an external emotional triggering event – his friend changing his plans at the last minute – which then started the emotional chain of events. It brings up negative feelings he has about himself, it further undermines his self-concept and lowers his self-esteem. Graham's planned emotional overeating is his revenge on himself for how and what he feels, which is useless and worthless. He was let down by his friend in what Graham perceived as a very dismissive manner, but he turned this incident inwards on himself. Graham has negatively internalised the external situation.

The Mini Moment Intervention is a useful and important strategy, which will help you stop any instant, and up until now seemingly uncontrollable, urges to eat when something highly distressing happens. You will take a look at what to do when the physical urge to eat occurs, how to help control it and what to do with it. This will be one of the most important techniques you will learn from *Stop Overeating*, because once you can stop any nutritionally unnecessary eating, you will start to lose weight, gain control of your emotional responses and begin to feel less negative about yourself and your future.

These here-and-now tactics will help you to stop both the instant emotional eating urges and, if you are like Graham, the planned emotional eating. Like a lot of emotional eaters you may have a history of both types of emotional eating. They are not exclusive behaviours and they can sit very close to each other. You may at first instantly respond to an emotionally provoking event by eating then and there. You may also plan further emotional eating in response to the situation or encounter and the fact that you've let yourself down by eating already.

In The Moment

The exercise opposite is what I have called the Mini Moment Intervention. I have specifically created and designed it to stop your urge to emotionally eat as it happens. It is a strategy which takes just 10 minutes. The Mini Moment Intervention will stop any in-the-moment emotional eating and can effectively be applied to any planned emotional eating too. In a short space of time, you will give yourself a thoughtful, conscious and compassionate period to consider what is going on for you emotionally.

The Emotional Wave

When you get an urge to emotionally eat it is rather like a wave coming in on a beach. At its highest point, your initial internally felt emotions are like the peak of the wave. They are emotionally intense for a really brief time, but it may seem like hours or even days because you get caught up in the whole episode of emotionally eating, the chain of events. However, the intense period, the initial felt emotions, really does only last for a brief time, a few moments. Like the wave, your initial emotional feeling, leading to eating, will soon lose its power and strength, but as an emotional eater you do not often get to that point.

It takes a few hours, sometimes days, to psychologically understand your emotional response to a situation or encounter completely, which is perfectly normal. The Mini Moment Intervention helps to stop a situation turning into an emotional eating episode. You need to learn to let any emotionally provoking incident lose its intensity and influence. Remember you have endured what is probably a lifetime of emotional eating, so be a little patient with yourself and do not assume you are going to be accurately naming the causes of your emotional eating in an instant. But what you can do in an instant is know not to eat because of them and wait for the 'wave' to lose its intensity for just 10 minutes. Remember it will dissipate.

Everyone, no matter what the situation is, can afford to give themselves 10 minutes, even the most habitual and established emotional eaters can do this. Ten minutes is not so long that you end up ruminating over what has happened, which may have further diet-blowing consequences, but is long enough to carefully consider what is going on for you.

The Mini Moment Intervention

Step One

The Mini Moment Intervention invites you to step away from an emotional trigger and to identify your feelings and what has made you need to emotionally eat. When you feel yourself needing to emotionally eat – knowing that you want to eat to deal with your emotions rather than to satisfy your physical hunger – then try to find some quiet mental space, and even physical space if possible, to properly examine your feelings.

Step Two

You may find it useful to quickly apply the five Ws: What, Where, When, Who and Why in your Mini Moment Intervention. Who was involved, what happened and what did you feel, and when and where did it happen? This will give you some brief thoughts about why you have ended up in this position of wanting to emotionally eat.

Step Three

It would be a good idea to make some brief notes during or after your Mini Moment Intervention. If you try to store these facts in your head, chances are they will become too overwhelming, distorted and raw. By trying to remember them you could be adding to your emotional vulnerability by recalling the details of something that is psychologically damaging. As a rule our psyche is not designed to do that, so make a note of them and put them to one side so you can come back to them later on in the Maxi Effect Analysis. Your notes can be written down, put on your phone or emailed to yourself, anywhere that you can pick up topics and your thoughts about them, for the next part of this week's session.

It is important you undertake the Mini Moment Intervention analysis properly, because if you do not you may find yourself falling into a trap of simply delaying or postponing your emotional eating until later, 10 minutes later to be precise. It is really easy and understandable to do that, and after a lifetime's emotional eating it will take conscious thought about your instant responses and reactions. With dedication and practice you will find the Mini Moment Interventions get quicker, easier and more effective as you use them. You can do a Backward Step exercise in that time, or make notes of any eating habits which may be reoccurring.

In the Mini Moment Intervention you can do enough psychological work for you to start rationalising, countering and positively challenging any negative emotional messages you are hearing and perceiving. This is a crucial 10 minutes when you will be both stopping the consumption of food itself and spending time considering and starting to mentally process the causes of your urges to emotionally eat.

Also in the Mini Moment Intervention you will stop thinking about food in terms of comfort, suppression or punishment. Crucially, and it is really important to emphasise this point, this is not a simple diversion strategy that simply delays any emotional eating.

Case Study: Kate

'To begin with I didn't think that 10 minutes was anywhere near long enough to think about all the things that contribute to my emotional eating. When I think about what I have discovered in the previous sessions, quite how far my habits around food alone have established themselves, let alone all the other things in my life,

I thought I would need much more time. But when the next opportunity came when I felt I was likely to emotionally eat I started to apply the 10-minute technique.

'At work another colleague was having a dinner party and I was not invited. When I heard her talking about it I felt anxious because I felt like there was something wrong with me to be left out. I instantly wanted to comfort myself with food because of how I felt and as this is habitually what I always do in these situations. I was aware that a lot of negative, familiar and nasty emotions were coming up. I decided to take just 10 minutes out to stop and focus on preventing them getting a grip on me, stop thinking about the provoked emotions for too long and stop thinking about the causes constantly or obsessively. I reminded myself that I can return to look at causes in a bit more detail later if I want to, when I'm not so sensitive, or after I've eaten a sensible regular meal.

'The technique stopped me from going straight to the coffee shop near my office for a large blueberry muffin or three. Applying the 10 minutes also stopped me eating my lunch early, which I have often done in the past as it gives me an excuse to get another calorie-filled one later on. For a very brief moment I remained focused on the emotionally provoking situation, the colleague's dinner party, and rationalised that she was only inviting two other people from the office and couldn't invite everyone, and as I hardly know her why would she invite me anyway? I wouldn't

invite her to anything I did. It made me realise just how hypersensitive I am to these situations. I made a few notes so I could return to them later if I wanted to and that seemed to get me over the initial wave of emotions I felt when I first heard about the dinner party and felt left out.'

Kate, like most people who start the Mini Moment Intervention, did not think 10 minutes was going to be anywhere near enough time to analyse the causes of her emotional eating, which she is right about to some extent. However, it is enough time to stop the actual eating and enough time to think, even if it is just for a few moments, about the causes of it (her deep-rooted anxieties about there being something wrong, something defective about her and being left out because of it). Remember it is like a wave, and you just need to give yourself 10 minutes to endure its intense peak, because like the wave, the emotional intensity will pass. There may be other waves that follow, but they will not be as emotionally intense as the initial one.

When Kate did a 10-minute Mini Moment Intervention she could see that there were a lot of familiar feelings coming up that have impacted on her emotional eating in the past. By taking a few minutes to simply stop the automatic habitual reaction of eating to comfort herself, Kate is helping not to ruin her weight-loss plans, which in turn will give her something to reflect on positively. Also, and very importantly, Kate is starting to think about some of the underlying issues that have been maintaining her emotional eating for such a long time. Kate will undertake a more detailed analysis in the next part of this session, the Maxi Effect Analysis (see page 117).

Case Study: Frank

'Recently my girlfriend and I had a huge row over money. We never seem to have enough of it; all the time I can feel myself feeling more ashamed and inadequate. And because I can't stand feelings like this, and I'll do anything to make them go away, it's usually straight to the chip shop. But I applied the Mini Moment Intervention to stop and think about how I was feeling and thought about how familiar it is for me to instantly try to bury and hide my feelings. I know I've got to do more work to get to the bottom of things, but because I stopped myself from instantly going to the chip shop it gave me a little bit of time to start to think about my eating. I could focus on wanting to stop being someone who is not in control of how they feel, but more importantly stop being someone who is not in control of how and what they eat. It was really useful because I didn't go to the chip shop, I didn't gorge myself on chips and pies and for the first time in a long while I began to experience a feeling of achievement with my eating.'

The technique is not going to work perfectly every single time. But even if it works for some of the time to start with, it will give you an enormous sense of achievement, which you can recall and bring back to your conscious mind the next time an emotional eating urge happens. In other words you will have done it and will have a template of being successful, so you know you can do it again.

Case Study: Linda

'The other night both Rob and Jamie were being their usual horrible selves to me. I sometimes think it's a bit of a competition between them as to who can upset me the most. As much as I was really upset with what they were saying about me, instead of going straight to the kitchen and going through a whole packet of biscuits or two like I normally would, I went up to my bedroom and for few minutes thought about what had just happened. It doesn't feel nice to be spoken to like that, but it did make it a lot better to not have eaten hundreds of extra calories because of it. And even when I have eaten in the past, it doesn't change anything about how Rob and Jamie speak to me or how I feel. I've done the Mini Moment Intervention a few times now and every time I feel much more in control of how I respond to certain emotional situations. And I can already see the effect on my weight, which makes me feel better too.'

The Mini Moment Intervention can be used to both physically stop your eating and to give yourself a dedicated short period of time to consider and take on board some of the issues in your life that lead you to emotionally eat every time something distressing or upsetting happens. Each time is going to be slightly different, but there will be certain themes, repeated situations and reappearances of people who are causing you problems and having an effect on your life, diet and use of food.

You are always going to be your own best judge of what works for you once you start to apply the Mini Moment Interventions. Remember to listen to yourself – you have valuable and important things to say to yourself which should not be overlooked.

Part 2
The Maxi Effect Analysis

In the previous part of this session you learnt how to do Mini Moment Interventions, which can stop your emotional eating as soon as you feel the urge to eat. Now, you are going to learn an important long-term strategy which I have devised called the Maxi Effect Analysis. This is going to help you get right to the root of your emotional eating, to identify the causes of it. If the Mini Moment Intervention was like having a brief call to your therapist to stop your urges to emotionally eat, then the Maxi Effect Analysis is going to be like having full one-to-one therapy with your therapist. You'll investigate and see what, and who, has helped to turn you into an emotional eater, and just as importantly what and who maintains it now.

When you undertake a Maxi Effect Analysis you will be looking for and at a number of different things:

- **Themes**
  Kate's Maxi Effect Analysis will be used to illustrate the themes concept of emotional eating.
- **Acknowledgement**
  Next, you will learn to acknowledge what is going on for you both now and in the past. Frank's Maxi Effect Analysis will help you with this one.
- **Tolerating**
  You will explore and start to gain an understanding

of tolerating your feelings for a short time when you hear and receive any negative emotional message. Linda's Maxi Effect Analysis will show you how it has helped.

When you have had a situation or encounter that starts an emotional chain of events and you have worked through a Mini Moment Intervention on it, hopefully you will have made some brief notes. Even if you did not use a Mini Moment Intervention it is still very useful to make notes about the emotionally triggering situation that upset or distressed you, your thoughts about the external emotional triggers, what you felt, when it happened, who and what may have been the cause of it and the potential starting point of the chain of events. This information is what you will be using along with all the other discoveries and observations you have been making throughout *Stop Overeating* in this second part of this session.

Understanding the Best Thing to Do

It is understandable that the Maxi Effect Analysis is not the easiest thing, because when an emotional event has happened the last thing you want to do is return to it. It is uncomfortable to think about both the event and your emotional response to it. However, not returning to analyse what happened in the emotional chain of events, whether or not it turned into a full-blown emotional eating episode, is a large part of what has sustained your emotional vulnerability and subsequent emotional eating over the years. You need to give yourself proper thinking time and space to really see what, and who, is causing your emotional upset.

Allowing a specific dedicated time to think about yourself in a kind, compassionate, understanding and non-critical way is something which you are probably not too familiar with. It may make you feel awkward, a bit embarrassed and perhaps even self-indulgent. So it will help your progress to become familiar with these slightly awkward feelings – the embarrassment will lessen as you get used to the idea of considering yourself and your emotional needs more often than and above the needs of others. For some, overcoming the awkward and embarrassing feelings is a crucial part of the therapeutic process of stopping their emotional eating.

The Maxi Effect Analysis

Step One

The Maxi Effect Analysis is about giving yourself a dedicated but limited time period, usually about an hour each time, to consider what has gone on for you. You could do this every few days to begin with to get used to the analysis process, or you could set aside a specific time once a week. This is the minimum amount of time that you should have as a lengthier analysis time. Do the exercise in a quiet, undisturbed place. Turn off your phone and, if you need to, make your excuses and leave the house if it is too noisy. You are trying to replicate what it would be like in one-to-one therapy as practically as possible, so it should be just you and the Maxi Effect Analysis – your therapist.

Step Two

You may want to work with a few provoking encounters, whether they turned into an emotional eating episode or not, to do the analysis. If nothing has happened to you which is emotionally triggering or provoking, that is good and just leave it at that. Do not start to magnify regular, non-provoking situations into something they are not. Make sure you have read through the entire session and be ready to work through the three key topics for the Maxi Effect Analysis: **themes**, **acknowledgement** and **tolerating**.

If you feel that you are having lots of emotional eating urges, or are experiencing a high number of emotionally provoking external triggers, then you can increase how many times you undertake a Maxi Effect Analysis. Eventually you will gain a sufficient understanding of what is happening emotionally, namely what and who is the cause of your fragile self-concept, your low self-esteem and how you negatively feel about yourself, which makes you vulnerable to emotional eating.

It is likely that the same or similar situations and people are coming up over and over again each time you do a Maxi Effect Analysis, but just because they are coming up repeatedly do not be tempted to stop thinking about and considering them. In therapy, the same people, situations and scenarios are often thought about and discussed, and this bringing them to mind, considering them and how they affect you, will facilitate psychological and emotional change. This is because you are giving yourself vital contained and self-empathetic time to reflect and mentally process the causes of your emotionally provoking incidents. Although there may be a lot of repetition of contributing variables, the actual situations, encounters and people, and your emotional understanding of the whole situation and the contributors to it, can and will change. For example, what you found completely distressing and upsetting the first time will now have a different effect because you have gained valuable psychological insights and understanding as you have gone through the exercises in this book. You will find yourself feeling a lot less emotional the next time you consider a similar or new situation, and again the time after that.

However painful, distressing, confusing or just plain annoying it is to keep the provoking incident and those who contributed to it at the front of your thoughts here, you are doing it because keeping them there in the front of your mind and consciousness will allow you to do something about them. Otherwise, the danger is that they just become forgotten and never addressed, which up until now is exactly what they always have been.

Your Themes

When you consider your episodes of emotional eating, are there any themes to them? Do similar situations keep repeating themselves or do the same people keep coming up over and over again? Perhaps, like Kate, you have a theme of emotionally eating because you seek comfort in food. Do you have a theme of significant previous experiences both as a child and an adult which leave you constantly fearing rejection and abandonment by others? Eating for comfort has become a habit for Kate, a theme. Maybe, like Kate, you also have the theme of your belief that being an emotional eater is part of who you are, it is what you and others expect of you. Kate believes she cannot cope very well without food because she has never tried.

For the themes part of the Maxi Effect Analysis, think about and make a note of the times when you emotionally eat and think honestly about whether you are genuinely hungry or not. Genuine physical hunger and emotional eating are not exclusive to each other. The problem comes, however, when unlike genuine physical hunger you cannot reach a point where you have had enough to eat. With emotional eating, you will never be satisfied. No amount of food will ever be enough to deal with, take away or make your emotional issues better. You need to think about and consider any themes as to what or who comes up for you in relation to your episodes of emotional eating. As with all the exercises in *Stop Overeating*, this information is just for your eyes and thoughts only – you are not required to show it to anyone so you can be as honest as possible. You can always destroy, delete or throw it away afterwards if you want to.

The one theme which comes up for most emotional eaters is that of people in your life, the ones who have upset you, the ones you may have identified in the Backward Step Technique exercise or the Relationship Analysis you did in your first session. The theme of the specific person, or type of people, who have added to your low self-concept, your low self-esteem and lack of belief in yourself is important to recognise. How others make you feel about yourself is probably the one main and underlying reason you have become an emotional eater in the first place and why you stay one still.

Case Study: Kate (Themes)

'When I think back over the last few times I have either emotionally eaten or really wanted to, what has become clear to me is that there is a theme of me being scared and fearful of being left out of things, which I then try to comfort with food. I can see the situations at work, being left out of the colleague's cake, not being invited to the dinner party, are similar to each other in that they make me feel really panicky that I was being left out for whatever reason, and I eat to comfort that panic, that sense of rejection. Also there is a distinct theme when

it comes to visiting my own family. How the visit goes is always dependent on my sister's mood, especially at the moment because Emma's still very jealous about me getting married so everyone is treading on eggshells around her. When I'm there I still end up with that feeling of being left out of things, with the others all having conversations I don't know about. If I'm honest I always feel a bit of a spare part.

'Exploring these themes to my emotional eating in a Maxi Effect Analysis helped me properly identify them and helps me to see that I emotionally eat because I'm scared of being left out and rejected. This is linked to how I feel about myself, that I'm not good enough to be wanted, which in itself is linked to how I was treated and thought about in the past by my family. In lots of different emotional eating situations, thoughts about how my sister and my mum have treated me kept coming up over and over again, regardless of whether they had something to do with that particular situation.

'Looking at these themes was good because instead of just mindlessly emotionally eating and not really knowing why, because I am now familiar with repetitive themes of people that cause my emotional eating, I feel I have a choice not to turn to food for comfort every five minutes, which is helping me stay much more focused on my weight loss.'

You need to be able to look at themes as objectively as possible so you can then move on to doing something about them. See any themes for what they are, which in Kate's case was a lot to do with her sister's problems, which she has been unwittingly absorbing throughout her life. Explore any themes, see where your thoughts about them take you, so eventually you can challenge them and go forwards managing your emotional eating.

You may also come up with themes of *when* you emotionally eat – weekends are a particularly common time because you are not only increasing the likelihood of being with people, especially your family, at the weekend, but also it is a traditional social eating time as well. Or maybe you emotionally eat more at bed time, or just before a regular meal. It is good to make a note of it because you are at your most susceptible to emotional eating when your energy levels are at their lowest. And being aware of this will mean you can do something about it. So, if you know you have a potentially emotionally provoking situation coming up, eat something sensible before you get there, or make sure you take some less calorie-laden food with you. That way if the emotional wave's peak happens you have something which, along with the 10 minutes of the Mini Moment Intervention, should stop the high-calorific emotional eating.

You may have themes of what particular foods you eat. Perhaps you want really indulgent comforting foods. Perhaps you eat food you do not like because of your need to not get any pleasure from it to punish yourself. Make a note and explore them in your Maxi Effect Analysis time to see if, and why, you have any specific foods you crave.

This is all vital information to help you stop eating for purely emotional reasons.

Your Acknowledgements

When I talk about acknowledgement this is in terms of identifying and acknowledging how you have been treated and thought about by others in your life. I want to make it clear that acknowledgement is not the same as acceptance and forgiveness. A lot of people get acknowledgement, acceptance and forgiveness mixed up, but they are completely different psychological concepts. You may have been treated appallingly in the past, and that is not right, but what is also not right is to let those experiences define you, keeping you attached to that time and susceptible to emotional eating. *Stop Overeating* is not about promoting acceptance and forgiveness, it is about finding ways for you to stop your emotional eating. One of those ways is going to be acknowledging what goes on for you, identifying what happens in your head, bringing everything into the open in this part of the session in a contained way, even if it is just you and a piece of paper.

For the acknowledgement part of the exercise, when thinking about anything which has come up during *Stop Overeating*, are there topics, people and places which, up to this point in your life, have not been properly identified and need to be acknowledged for what they are, like Kate's work colleague and family, Frank's mother's actions or Linda's partner and family's attitude? Maybe you want to acknowledge how you have been treated by your family, or how your friends have behaved towards you. It is anything at all that you have found upsetting or distressing enough to have to emotionally eat because of. This may be something which is inconsequential to others, even to those directly involved, but it is the complete opposite for you.

There may be only one or two important things for you to acknowledge or there may be lots, but acknowledging them and the harm they have done to you and your emotional eating will help you move on from them. If they continue to smoulder on unacknowledged in your thoughts and psyche it will very likely cause further upset and distress and will lead to subsequent emotional eating. Acknowledging could be about making a list, mental or written down, of all the people in your past and present who you honestly and genuinely feel have caused you emotional upset. Again this is just for your eyes and thoughts.

Do not take any more than five minutes to do this exercise. You do not want to spend too long on it as it is likely that the same people will come up repeatedly. The acknowledgement task is about giving you a chance to properly acknowledge the damage and harm that others have caused you and – this is the crucial bit – once you have made that acknowledgement you can then move on, or at least start to find some psychological distance from things. Start by looking at your most recent emotional eating episode and note down the person and the emotion associated with it. They may not have been present or even directly involved, but the fact that you are making an association between them, the incident and your emotions is important to acknowledge. It is not about continually blaming people for what and why you emotionally eat and using them as an excuse. It is about properly acknowledging them so you can move on, leaving them and their emotionally toxic legacy behind you at last.

Case Study: Frank (Acknowledgement)

'Although my mum didn't set out to neglect me or not care for me when I was younger, the fact that she did has been something that it has taken me a long time to comes to terms with. I can see how being in denial about this has affected my eating and whole relationship with food for as long as I can remember. For whatever reason, Mum has always found it hard to really think about anyone but herself and I've been making a lifetime of excuses for her. But how she behaved, with the boyfriends, the drink and her neglect of me was wrong. She could have got a lot more help for me. And because I was very quiet and fairly resourceful when I was young, apart from the one horrible time in a children's home, I think I always managed to stay off any authority's radar. No one really took any notice of me at school and because that is what I was used to at the time, it didn't seem so unusual. But now I have my own children I can see that this was not right. Someone should have been looking out for me.

> *'I don't blame Mum for how she was towards me,
> she was a kid herself, but looking at the importance of
> acknowledgements in the Maxi Effect Analysis, I was
> able to acknowledge that it has had an effect on how
> I feel about myself. I still struggle to believe that I'm a
> worthwhile person to care about. I also acknowledge that
> because feeling I'm not worthwhile or important is such a
> painful thing to think about, I've been covering it up and
> avoiding it for years with food.*
>
> *'Emotional eating has been my instant default
> setting when anything remotely confrontational has
> come up, both in the past and right now. Being able to
> acknowledge how I really feel about myself now (not just
> why I eat) and who has been the origin and the main
> cause of it, Mum, has been hugely beneficial. I know that
> she won't change her attitude towards how she treated
> me when I was a child. But I can acknowledge that she
> won't, and I can change my own attitude. I do not have
> to be that little boy who uses food to hide behind all the
> time any more.'*

Remember, acknowledging what and who has affected you in the past, and has the potential to in the future, is going to be another vital tool to stopping and managing your emotional eating. Acknowledgement will allow you to move on. Frank is acknowledging how he feels about himself and what he feels is the original cause of his emotional eating – his mother, which will be beneficial to stopping it. He is no longer in a never-ending cycle of emotionally eating – he has a way to break the cycle and lose weight successfully.

Some people I have worked with in the past have found this a very difficult exercise to complete and implement. They were not ready to let go of their psychological and emotional status and move on. It will take a lot of personal challenge and resilience to change being stuck, because if you acknowledge and change your thoughts and attitude you will have to change other things in your life too: the amount you eat or what you eat; you may need to change your job, or get a job; lose all the secondary gains you looked at in the Beliefs of an Emotional Eater section in Session Two. Without change you will simply and unhappily stay a victim of your past and your circumstances and you will remain very susceptible to emotional eating because of it.

Acknowledging what has gone on for you in the past, and indeed still goes on for you now, which has caused your emotional eating can be extremely difficult. If you are finding it too upsetting, because you are thinking about things which have been buried by food for many years, just do it at a pace that suits you. You can carry on with the rest of the book and come back to this if you need to.

Your Tolerance

Next you are going to learn how to tolerate and cope during those highly emotive moments, the peak of the emotional wave moments that have you heading straight for the food cupboard. Learning to tolerate your provoked negative emotional message is going to be unusual, if not a little difficult to begin with. Knowing that it is possible to hold on to and contain certain unwelcome feelings, even for a short while, until the peak of the wave goes away, will be another helpful and important tool to stopping being an emotional eater. Tolerating is having the mental capacity to hold on to how you feel at any one emotionally provoking moment so you do not automatically and emotionally eat. Understanding how to properly tolerate is a really crucial tool to stopping you emotionally eating, supporting the work you began to do in the Mini Moment Intervention.

When you use the Mini Moment Intervention, it is about the here-and-now moment. In the Maxi Effect Analysis it is about thinking about all the different situations and people who have contributed to how you feel about yourself and being able to hold on to that. In other words to tolerate and build up the mental capacity to deal with those emotional moments by not turning to food the instant the negative thoughts and feelings emerge. To start with, tolerating will probably be almost unnatural and will go against everything your thoughts and behaviour want to do. But remember that acting on that impulse is the very thing which has contributed to you being overweight. In psychotherapy, when we talk about toleration it can mean so many things. Tolerating thinking about certain things and people is something you did in the Acknowledgement part of this exercise. Tolerating being in the moment with yourself, however unusual and uncomfortable it is, just giving yourself the space and time to think, is going to be really beneficial and useful to you.

People become emotional eaters because they cannot stand the highly emotive moment they find themselves in. They cannot tolerate the horrible feelings, they find it unbearable to think and feel the way they do about themselves or those close to them, especially if those close to them are the original trigger to the emotional eating episode. So they turn to food to take those unwelcome and unwanted feelings away – to bury them, to ignore them, anything at all that stops them thinking about the meaning and cause of them. However, not only are they not doing their health and waistline any good, they are not doing their psychological health any good either, and it will only get worse. A major part of overcoming and managing your emotional eating will be about learning how to tolerate those horrible feelings, even if it is just briefly enough so you do not go to the food cupboard. Learning to tolerate what comes up emotionally is like an extended version of the Mini Moment Intervention, with more psychological and psychoanalytical depth, and most importantly with a compassion and tolerance towards yourself you probably have not experienced before.

Learning to tolerate your emotions when an emotionally provoking situation or encounter happens will need practice. So rather than wait for the next situation or encounter to come along you can help yourself by thinking about past emotional eating episodes and what your feelings were if you can recall them. It is often useful to go back to your most recent episodes of emotional eating or choose a particularly significant episode of emotional eating which stands out for you, maybe a family Christmas, a romantic date or a job interview. Try to remember how you felt, look at the negative emotions list on page 31 to help identify the emotions and then just practise holding on to them. Recall how you feel and felt mentally for a few seconds. The feelings that have re-emerged will go, like the wave, so take a few deep breaths until they subside. This is not going to be the same as a real emotionally provoking moment, but it will be a good starting point to practise tolerating your feelings so when a new situation or encounter does happen you are practised, rehearsed and ready for it.

If you find that it is getting too stressful or difficult, remind yourself it is a past event, it is gone and that the emotional eating damage, if there was any on that occasion, has been done. What you are trying to do is just practise holding on to how you felt in a way you can control. If you fear going back to previous emotionally provoking experiences because you worry that you will end up mentally and emotionally stuck there, it may be a good idea to schedule in something that cannot be broken afterwards, even if it is just watching a favourite TV programme, keeping an appointment or meeting or contacting friends. Anything at all so you do not get mentally stranded in the past when you do any practising.

Like anything worthwhile it is essential to practise tolerating your emotional response, even if it is for a very short time, because when the actual situation or encounter happens you will need to know that you can indeed tolerate it and have the mental capacity to hold on to any provoked emotions in a way which is not going to be harmful.

Case Study: Linda (Tolerance)

'Practising tolerating the horrible feelings I get after any upsetting episode while doing the Maxi Effect Analysis was a little difficult to start with. I really didn't want to recall times when I'd been so emotionally overwhelmed that I ended up eating because of them. But I challenged myself and remembered a recent and significant episode, when both Rob and Jamie were really nasty to, and about, me. Jamie started going on about not being given enough money to buy things and Rob was being just Rob, nasty and hateful towards me and egging Jamie on. As ever I'd ended up in the kitchen eating a whole double packet of plain chocolate digestives, which I don't even particularly like.

'Focusing on what I felt at that time was unusual to begin with – it had been just another one of so many familiar times. But when I started to think about how I felt, surprisingly it was quite easy because the feelings were very familiar: that I'm useless because I can't do the things other people want me to – can't have enough money for Jamie and be a proper partner for Rob. Even after 15 years together I don't know what he wants from me, but whatever it is I do know that I *don't give it to him. But I practised a little bit of deep breathing and thought about what was going on there. Jamie is behaving like a spoilt brat, which sadly is nothing new, and Rob, well, he's behaving just like my father: dismissive, demanding and fickle.*

'It was a real wake-up moment for me. I realised that their behaviours don't always have to affect mine quite so much. I also thought about other, all-too-familiar, emotionally provoking times, usually to do with Jamie and Rob. Painful as it was to bring them back up again, it gave me a chance to let how I felt at the time stay with me, not automatically be buried or hidden under yet another packet of biscuits, giant chocolate bar or family-sized bottle of diet cola. Just letting these emotions sit with me for a few minutes and not instantly turning to food was both very unusual and strangely satisfying.

'Today a similar situation arose: Jamie was demanding new football boots calling me all sorts of things because I said I couldn't afford them and Rob was egging him on again. But I didn't react in my usual way. I got upset, of course, but instead of heading to the kitchen I went upstairs instead to watch the TV. On my way upstairs I was thinking about what had gone on and then watched TV while the emotional wave lost its power. For the first time I can remember, because I didn't give in to how I felt and eat, I felt proud of myself.'

Tolerating what is happening emotionally is going to be a key tool in stopping and managing your emotional eating when something happens to you which is unpleasant, scary or just plain nasty. Linda has learnt that, by holding on to the moment at the end of the emotional chain of events where the negative emotional message comes through for a few moments, instead of heading to the kitchen to block it out, she can use the new tactic of tolerating it for a short while. Just because she is holding on to the message, it does not mean that she is agreeing with, or accepting it. What is really important is that Linda is not harming her self-concept even further by eating, or lowering her self-esteem because of the message. Also she is giving herself valuable thinking space and time to examine things. If it is ever too emotive to do, Linda can come back to it later when she is less emotional and more logical if she wants to analyse it further.

In the Maxi Effect Analysis you have been learning how to identify themes, practise acknowledgement and apply tolerating to yourself. Some of these features may be more pertinent to you than others. What is appropriate and significant may change from one Maxi Effect Analysis to another. This is the nature of therapy and you will experience and bring different things to your therapy space (the Maxi Effect Analysis) so you can use it as appropriately and as usefully as you need. If something is more important one time then think about it and reflect on it. Remember, as in traditional one-to-one therapy you take what you explore, think about, acknowledge and reflect on with you to apply during the rest of your week. When I see people for therapy I remind them that we meet for an hour each week and they have to use what they think about and we discuss in that time for the other 167 hours until we meet again. It is not just about being in the room with me that counts or where all the work is done and the progress made. Clients do the bulk of stopping their emotional eating, understanding what and who is behind it, by themselves. With all the work you have been doing in *Stop Overeating*, all the discoveries and observations you have made, all the changed ways of thinking and adopting a new and healthier attitude about yourself, you are doing the same.

In the final part of this week's session you will learn the techniques and strategies to at last properly challenge any negative emotional messages, which, up until now, have been so damaging to your self-concept and how you feel about yourself.

Part 3
Challenging

Identifying themes and acknowledging and tolerating your emotional responses are all valuable and important tools towards managing your emotional eating. However, if you want to stop your emotional eating for good so you can diet successfully and retain your weight loss, you are going to need learn how to challenge any negative emotional messages you experience at the end of the emotional chain of events. By getting into the routine of challenging and properly investigating them from the first time you hear or receive the message, it will stop the message from escalating and increasing in magnitude and damage. Just because you feel and experience a certain emotion, or cluster of emotions, and then receive the subsequent negative emotional message, you do not have to necessarily agree with it or accept it.

You have got used to thinking about yourself in a certain way, which any negative emotional message latches on to, but that does not make the message authentic, valid or correct at all. You have probably had a lifetime's exposure to hearing and receiving the negative emotional message. It is hardly surprising that you have undoubtedly built up a reluctant resignation to it. The negative emotional messages have found an easy home in your thoughts and self-concept.

Perhaps because of the negative emotional messages you have been receiving over the years, which have all been chipping away at your self-esteem, you may have even found yourself agreeing with the people who say that if you ate less and worked out more you would not have any weight problems. In other words, being overweight is a simple formula of eating too much and exercising too little. Every emotional eater would love that simple formula to be true because then they could just stop eating without anything else in their lives influencing it. But as emotional eaters know, it is never going to be that simple. If it was, then you, me and every other emotional eater around would have done it ages ago.

Challenging Your Negative Emotional Messages

Even if you are applying the Mini Moment Intervention strategies and Maxi Effect Analysis tolerance technique, you will still need to learn how to challenge, investigate and dismiss the negative emotional messages for the long term.

You are going to take on the task of investigating, disputing and ultimately dismissing any negative emotional messages you receive and hear from the emotions you experience. Unlike the many complex and intricate reasons for emotional eating, this technique is quite simple and straightforward. As soon as you hear the negative emotional messages, whatever they are, you need to start to question them, cross-examine them, consider any alternative explanation for them, and ask if there is any supporting evidence for them if you really do believe them. There is unlikely to be any supporting evidence for your negative emotional message, so do not start embellishing or twisting evidence to support it unnecessarily. As odd as it may seem, I have treated people who have done this to some degree or another for varied reasons, such as a resistance to thinking about themselves differently or having a reluctance to believe they can change their perceptions of others in their lives. It can also be about a reluctance to want to make the changes to their diet and exercise that they know they will have to adopt.

Challenge

Step One

What you are going to do in this Challenge exercise is to go back to the Statement of Feelings exercise (page 41) to retrieve the original negative emotional messages. As you have got this far in *Stop Overeating* and the original emotional chain of events you worked on may be many days, weeks or even months ago, it would be fine to use a more up-to-date Statement of Feelings exercise and note down the negative emotional messages from it. Now, take those three Statements of Feeling – the negative emotional messages – and analyse, challenge and dismiss them in a rational and well-judged way.

Step Two

How you challenge the negative emotional messages is going to be up to you. Some people like to write them down to challenge them, others like to verbalise them to dispute them. Some people will do a combination of both writing and verbalising – you need to find out what works for you best. Different situations and encounters will require different responses; it is going to be whatever suits you at the time. It is best if you can do this as close to the received negative emotional message as possible. Remember, you have your Mini Moment Intervention strategy to help in the actual moment to ensure that you are not eating, so you can come back to the proper analytical challenging a little later if you want to.

If You Need a Little Help

You might not feel confident enough to take on the role of examiner to start with when doing this exercise, and it is very useful to perhaps have an advocate in mind who can help. You do not actually get that person to do any of the questioning of your negative emotional message, they do not even know about it, rather you just imagine them doing it for you. Perhaps it could be someone genuinely supportive from the Relationship Analysis exercise you did in Session One. Or, choose a strong, sympathetic well-known person, someone you feel would really challenge the negative emotional message on your behalf. Whichever type of person you choose, you simply ask yourself the question, *'What would so and so say to these negative emotional messages I am receiving if they were here?'* It might seem strange at first to imagine someone standing up to your negative emotional message, but it is the start of really doing something about them for the first time. Often, once you get into the habit of challenging any negative emotional message via a third party advocate in your head, your own voice will soon emerge in its own right. In other words it is you and you alone who will be challenging your negative emotional message. Using someone known to you as an advocate is what we psychologists call a 'fake it until you make it' approach, which lots of people have found really helpful, especially at the beginning of challenging their negative emotional messages. If you feel at all silly or uncomfortable by employing this tactic, remember that absolutely no one but you has to know about your advocate as they are in your thoughts alone.

Whichever strategy you choose to use, it may change for different negative emotional messages. You will need to ask a few questions of the actual negative emotional message, questions such as: *'What is the evidence to support that view I have of myself?'* or *'Is someone else's personal agenda being played out and reflected in my negative emotional message?'* or *'Am I being emotionally used or dumped on by someone else?'* or *'Am I gaining in any way from accepting and agreeing with the negative emotional message?'* Remember the Secondary Gain belief you looked at in the Beliefs of an Emotional Eater in Session Two for this final question.

If you get stuck on what may be the answer to any of your cross-examinations of the negative emotional message, go back to the emotional trigger Backward Step exercise and look at the situation and encounters that started off the whole emotional chain of events. Look to see if there is anything or anyone in the Backward Step who is not only responsible for the start of the emotional chain of events – you already know that – but can be highlighted and labelled as someone who is also responsible for how you have ended up feeling about yourself. When you do the Challenge exercise, what you are aiming for is a modest shift, especially at the beginning, in how you feel about yourself. It does not have to be a huge psychological change to start with. As you become familiar with the exercise, the change in your feelings about yourself will continue and increase, as will your confidence and self-esteem. Let's follow Kate, Frank and Linda through this exercise for guidance and examples of applying the Challenge technique.

Case Study: Kate

'When I wrote my original negative emotional messages down from the Understanding the Emotional Chain of Events session to analyse, they were: **"I'm not worth caring about." "I'm invisible, not worth taking notice of." "There's so much wrong with me."** I really did not have the confidence to set about challenging them by myself, so I imagined what my best friend Sara, who I've known since childhood and who is very honest and truthful with me, would say to them. Sara has known Emma for years so knows what she is like – attention-seeking, manipulating.

'So I imagined Sara standing next to me cross-examining these negative messages, demanding on what basis they stand there in my thoughts, influencing me. The ones about me being worthless and invisible were challenged first, and it was good because instantly I could come back and write down that I'm not worthless or invisible to my husband, he really loves and cares for me, and his family too. I know my parents love and care for me, but they are so wrapped up in Emma all the time it's hard to feel that. But that's their choice, I can't do anything about it, so I don't have to keep letting it affect me as much. Applying the Acknowledgement technique helped here.

'Then it came to the third statement of how I feel, the negative message of **"There's so much wrong with me."** Again imagining Sara there being my advocate, I wrote down that yes, I know that I'm not perfect, none of us are, but it really doesn't have to lead to thinking that everything is wrong with me, because it is not. I have a loving husband, supportive friends. There's lots going on in my life that, if not fantastically wonderful, is really okay and I need to be more aware of it.

'From the observations and information I have discovered from the previous sessions and exercises, I know that Emma, and how she acts towards other people as well as me, has been a big contributor to how I feel about myself, not just for this particular episode of emotional eating, but throughout a lot of my life. I had not realised to what extent she had been influencing how I feel about myself. I will do something about her in my thoughts and attitude, even if I never get to saying anything to her, which to be honest she would just try to turn around and create more drama about, playing the victim to my persecutor. But I will change my attitude towards her. I have to, otherwise for the immediate future she's going to be negatively affecting me and I really don't want that for both our sakes.

'Also when I really started to look at the situation with the work colleague and her cake, she's the one with the problem. She got transferred because she cannot do the job she was employed to do, and although she's rotten to me, she would be to anyone who was brought in to replace her. I have plenty of friends in the office who I know value me, because they would not ask me to go out with them outside of work otherwise. It's amazing how one person and her cake, which some of my friends *brought over to me, can have such a devastating, but completely unjustified, effect. And I'm determined to not let it happen again.'*

Although many people are emotional eaters, the fact is, like for Kate, there are so many different circumstances and influences to each individual emotional eating episode, let alone each individual person, so any episode of emotional eating is going to be completely unique to you. Without exception, each emotional eater is different and every episode of emotional eating involves constantly changing variables, such as state of mind, circumstances, people, memories, time of day, time of month or time of year. They all subtly, and not so subtly, have made their contributions to your emotional eating. When it comes to emotionally eating, there is no 'one size fits all' category. We are too individual and too interesting for that and, as all the discoveries and observations you have been working on so far in *Stop Overeating* have told you, emotional eaters use food for many different reasons in their lives.

Case Study: Frank

'I know that I have been avoiding doing anything about my emotional eating for far too long, and when I looked at the negative emotional messages I got from the end of the Understanding the Emotional Chain of Events session they were not new to me. But I know that if I'm ever going to properly do something about my weight I have to really tackle and take them on. My received messages were

that **"I am damaged and flawed."** That **"I'm no use, I can't provide and am not good enough."** That **"I'm a coward and can't face my responsibilities."** I know that I'm no good at arguing, after all I've been running away from any confrontation all my life. So I had to think about someone who I admire and who I thought would be a good supporter of me if they were here.

'There's a player in the England football team who I've always admired – he always seems pretty straightforward and upfront about things when interviewed, he says it like it is. So I thought about what it would be like to have him standing next to me confronting these nasty, but familiar messages. On the first one that **"I am damaged and flawed"**, as I have been exploring through the exercises in the book, I really did not have a very secure, let alone happy, childhood. In fact if I could sum it up in one word, surprisingly it wouldn't be the word "eating", it would be "anxious". I was always so scared of being taken away again, and Mum just didn't seem to ever want to do anything about it, either the situation itself or my anxiety about it. So perhaps it's not unexpected that I have come out of it feeling like this. But just because I have had that sort of upbringing it does not have to continue to make me damaged and flawed, which acknowledging helped me to see. I have a great girlfriend, and I know my boys love me. If I were as damaged as I often think I am, they wouldn't love me or want to be with me.

'When my advocate and I moved on to cross-examine the second statement that **"I'm no use, I can't provide**

and am not good enough", *it wasn't too long before I started to think about finances being hard at the moment for everyone, not just me. I should be more responsible by not going to the fast food places and getting takeaways all the time. My uncle does offer me as much work as he's got, and again if I were not good enough, as I let myself believe, he wouldn't. So when I can I do provide, although I do have to do something about the fast food because it's bad for my waistline and wallet in so many ways.*

'When I examined the third message **"I'm a coward and can't face my responsibilities"**, *I thought that life is always going to be about having to deal with troubling things. Although I have to admit it's been a real pain to not deal with them, it does have its benefits. I have been eating whatever I wanted to for such a long time, but I know I have to stop. I can't keep using what happens with my mum as a reason, I need to face some responsibilities. I'm not a bad person, I just happen to have been brought up by someone who was, for whatever reason, uncaring, and I know it has had an effect on me. Any negative messages seem to home straight in to my thoughts, how I feel about myself. But I'm an adult man now; I can make my own choices. I know my mother will always play a part in my life in one way or another, but I can make the decision and have the control so that it doesn't always have to be so damaging.'*

Because you have been hearing the negative emotional messages for most of your life you have got used to accepting them and agreeing with them for one reason or another. Quite often the emotional messages are rooted in a very basic survival technique for a lot of people. Frank had a neglectful childhood, but if he had tried to challenge how he was being treated and the associated negative emotional message he received from that treatment, it could have ended very badly for him: Frank had already had one unpleasant time in a children's home and was fearful of it being repeated.

Remember when you do this exercise that you are aiming for a discreet and modest shift in how you feel about yourself. It does not have to be a huge change to start with, but as long as there is some kind of movement that is what is important.

Case Study: Linda

"Everything wrong is my fault." "I'm weak and stupid." "I don't deserve anything better." *Even though these particular negative emotional messages were my most recent, if I'm honest I've been hearing them in one form or another since I can remember. The first thing I wanted to do was see if I could challenge them by myself. It would be good to imagine an advocate being with me, and there are a few people I can think of, including my friend at work and a breakfast TV presenter who always seems to be genuinely caring and interested in people and their problems. But I wanted to do the challenge on my own.*

'For the first message, **"Everything wrong is my fault."**, I've been feeling that everything is all my fault for years, and that perhaps I have made a contribution to things not being right with Rob, Jamie and Dad. But when I start to look at any evidence for this statement, it really is not true. Jamie is sadly choosing to be like his dad, which perhaps is hardly surprising as it's all he's ever known, but when Rob's not around he can still be very sweet and nice to me. Maybe I need to tell him how much his actions and words affect me. If I look at all three of them together, Jamie's behaviour is the one that most bothers me. Rob and Dad have been telling me that everything wrong is my fault for years, but I do not have to believe their version of me, because there is nothing to support it. A lot of it is them dumping on me: Dad for me not being a boy, Rob for not being, well, everything. But these are Rob's issues not mine. I've been doing my best for years with Jamie and Dad, earning regular money, which is more than Rob has ever done. Everyone has their choices in life and Dad's and Rob's have, without doubt, affected mine. And even if it just stays in my head for the time being, tolerating it, I do not have to agree to be the person they tell me I am.

'It is the same for feeling **"weak and stupid"**. I may have been giving in to one man or another for as long as I can remember, often for very practical reasons, but I do not have to agree with this statement. I may not be the most qualified person in the world, but I have many other attributes, like being caring, truthfulness, loyalty to *my boss – lots of positive things that get so buried under all the negatives. It takes a mental effort because it is so unusual to focus on my positives.*

*'The final negative message, **"I don't deserve anything better"** is quite easy to challenge because who doesn't deserve better? I may have some flaws and deficits, but it doesn't mean I don't deserve to feel happy and loved. Regardless of what Dad and Rob may say, which I've been believing for far too long, I do deserve as much as anyone else in life. I'm not a bad person, I've just made some bad choices.'*

An Easy Alternative

Some people have found taking on the challenge of their negative emotional message a little too difficult and unsatisfactory to begin with, so I have devised a simpler, quicker version of challenging your negative emotional messages. All you need to do is to reverse the original statement of the received negative emotional message and add why this reversed statement is true. So, taking a look at Kate's, Frank's and Linda's first negative emotional messages as an example, for Kate her first message would be *'I am worth caring about because ...'* For Frank his first negative emotional message statement reversed would be something like *'I am a good person, all things considered, because ...'* Linda's first negative emotional message statement would be *'It's not my fault because ...'* To complete your own reversed statements, think about all the things about you that are positive, constructive and good. The list of positive attributes opposite may help you. Choose those that reflect your own strengths. If you need to, get your envisaged advocate to help give you a positive character reference. It could be anything at all, it does not necessarily have to be a huge change of self-opinion, it can be a modest change in thought or a discreet shift in how you feel about yourself.

Kate reversed her negative emotional message to read *'I am worth caring about because ... I know I'm reliable and independent. I am a good friend to have because I'm helpful and honest.'* For Frank, his first negative emotional message reversed would be something like *'I am a good person, all things considered, because... despite what has happened to me when I was younger I'm still trusting, honest and very loyal to those around me.'* Linda's first negative emotional message statement turned around would read *'It's not my fault because ... of everything and all those around me that causes me emotional stress. In spite of them I'm dependable, I'm still a very genuine person and, despite the best efforts of those around me, I am reliable.'*

This is a chance to point out, highlight and remind yourself of your attributes and positive character traits. In all my years of therapy I have yet to find anyone who did not have something good and positive to say about themselves, no matter how small and however unwilling they have been to name them out loud. And self-attribution and self-affirmation are usually the last things on any emotional eater's list. Any attributes and skills have usually remained hidden and buried under a mountain of negative emotional messages and personal circumstances for such a long time.

Positive Attributes

Able	Genuine
Accepting	Good-humoured
Adequate	Good-natured
Admirable	Graceful
Agreeable	Happy
Alert/Awake	Helpful
Amenable	Hope/Hopeful
Assured	Important
Astute	Independent
Authentic	Intelligent
Believable	Interesting/Interested
Calm	Joyous
Capable	Likable
Confident	Lovable
Content	Not to be faulted
Credible	Positive
Defendable	Powerful
Dependable	Resilient
Effective	Secure
Empathetic	Significant
Forthcoming	Straightforward
Free	Strong
Friendly	Successful

Tolerant	Wanted
Understood/	Worthwhile
Understanding	Worthy
Valuable	

In this part of the Start to Stop session you have worked hard to accurately and properly challenge the negative emotional messages you receive and hear. The negative emotional message is something which has the potential to always be around in one form or another in most people's lives, whether they are emotional eaters or not. Having the techniques and strategies to be able to challenge them is crucial in dismissing and rejecting what are essentially highly prejudicial untruths about yourself, which is an essential part of stopping your emotional eating for good.

session 4 / week 4
Moving Beyond Emotional Eating

Introduction

There are no exercises to do in this final session. Instead you will be exploring three aspects of emotional eating that may impede and stop your weight-loss and diet plans:

1. Saboteurs
2. FOMO – Fear of Missing Out
3. Allowance days

These problems have been identified by many people undergoing therapy for emotional eating as having potential damaging and harmful effects on them, and as factors which they had not previously been aware of or taken into account.

Saboteurs operate on many different psychological levels, consciously or subconsciously, blatantly or subtly, but what they all do is to try to sabotage your already difficult dieting efforts because of a perceived threat your weight loss poses to their own psychological integrity, their sense of self, their way of life. Saboteurs will do almost anything to maintain your weight or increase your diet failure to reduce any psychological threat to themselves from your success.

In the second part of this session you will examine 'FOMO', which stands for Fear Of Missing Out – the acute panicky and anxious feelings you get when the type of food you want to eat is being denied you, usually because of your diet.

Finally, you will take a look at the concept of 'allowance days', the type of days – which often turn into weeks and months – where something goes wrong and you end up seeking and eating unhealthy foods. You eat for the sake of eating – your emotional eating in its most basic form.

It is hard enough starting and staying on a diet so if you can make it any easier for yourself by uncovering potential and hidden problem makers for you, then you will be in a far better place to succeed with your weight loss.

Part 1
Saboteurs

Case Study: Justine

'I have been trying to do something about being overweight for a good few months now. I make no secret of it at home, with friends or in the office. I want people to know so I can get as much support as possible. On the whole I am supported apart from by this one girl in our office.

'She wants to lose about the same amount of weight as I do and we informally started our diets together. However, right from the start she suddenly began to bring food into work, which she'd never done before. At first it was bags of crisps, peanuts, biscuits or chocolates, saying it was because she was clearing out her cupboards for her diet. But then she started to bring in cakes, doughnuts, pastries, all the things you'd actually have to buy. She says it's for everyone, but oddly enough all this food always seems to be put next to me on my desk, or next to my salad in the fridge. If I do lose even a tiny bit of weight she has to know about it, commenting on my clothes being baggy, or my face being slimmer and how I need to stop dieting. It's only ever a couple of pounds at the most, so I know it doesn't make that much difference.

'She'll say in a half-joking way that she doesn't want to be the only fat one in the office. She hasn't got on

> *at all well with her diet, and because of all the things*
> *she's been bringing in (which I have told her I have a*
> *weakness for) neither have I. It's hard enough being on*
> *a diet without having all the food I crave being wafted*
> *around in front of me. It was only when another friend in*
> *the office pointed out that she's been feeding me very*
> *subtly all this time that I realised what she's been doing*
> *to sabotage my diet.'*

As Justine says, when you start trying to do something about your weight it can be really hard work, even without any emotional eating issues. It is going to be made even harder if you then have to recognise, counter and deal with the diet-sabotaging actions of others too. You might encounter potential saboteurs while you undertake your weight loss who try to stop it, as well as trying to make you regain weight once you have lost it. You may meet saboteurs infrequently or you may have one in your life constantly. Either way, they cause havoc and harm to your good intentions and are determined to stop you succeeding in losing weight.

Whatever the reason – and there are many – for consciously or subconsciously sabotaging your weight-loss attempts, it is done because of a perceived threat and risk by your weight loss to the saboteur themselves and their own psychological integrity. This could be a threat to their own self-concept or the perception of a risk to their way of life. They will often see your weight loss as a threat to their fragile sense of self, a threat to their role, a threat to their control, all of which manifests itself in a sense of unacknowledged inadequacy, which is then in turn played out and projected at you. The saboteur will do almost anything to maintain your weight and increase the likelihood of your diet failing because it then reduces any psychological threat to themselves resulting from your success. Saboteurs are really only interested in keeping your self-concept unchanged or lowered to maintain or increase their own.

This may all sound very intricate and convoluted, but it is one of the main reasons why so many people, without really realising it, slowly give up on their diet.

The actual sabotaging itself can take on different forms, the most frequent being jealousy, ignorance, scepticism and superiority. Remember the primary aim of a saboteur is to stop you doing what you want to do. It may be weight loss this time, it maybe something completely unrelated like moving home or getting a new job next time, but they want to stop you doing it, or make it as difficult as possible, because of the threat to their self-concept, integrity and way of life if you succeed at it.

In the following pages you will briefly explore some of the different types of saboteurs there are so you know what their thoughts, actions and behaviours are likely to be. Once you know them you can be ready for them, and not let them ruin your weight-loss plans or weaken your motivation to succeed.

The Jealous Saboteur

Saboteurs become jealous for many reasons, some obvious, some not so obvious. The fact that you are trying to do something decisive about your weight issues is a very common reason for jealousy to manifest itself in sometimes unexpected people in your life. As Justine said of her office feeder: *'she doesn't want to be the only fat one in the office.'* However, what she did not add to that statement was that she did not want Justine to be the slim one, the one who succeeded when she did not, and she will do anything she can to stop it, hence the endless amounts of food that Justine has a particular weakness for being brought in. All saboteurs are potentially dangerous to your diet, but ones with such a fixed agenda like this can be particularly threatening.

Often the jealousy is a deep-rooted and long-standing psychological insecurity that is played out and projected on to you. The exact reason why the person is jealous of your diet efforts and threatened by the anticipated success of your diet is in many ways irrelevant. However, you have got to consider your psychological wellbeing, your emotions, your physical welfare and your weight more than theirs. If someone is jealous of your attempts or commitment to lose weight and is prepared to sabotage your efforts because of it, do not be dragged in. Even if you do give in, it will not make them stop. If anything it will encourage them more because the less weight-loss success you have, the more psychological success they have.

The Ignorant Saboteur

When it comes to food, we tend to be either a Take It or a Leave It type of eater. As someone who has weight problems you are going to be a Take It type, as all emotional eaters tend to be. It really is not fair that you are this type of character, the type that cannot say no when the biscuits are passed around, who even if you do manage to say no wants to say yes.

Odd as it seems to us, the Take It type of eaters, there are people who are genuinely not that interested in food and eating – the Leave It type. These people honestly do not know what it is really like to find refusing food difficult. It is a bit like asking opposite sexes to know what it is like to be the other one. We have information and observations of them, we may even know a few of them personally, but we are not them, so cannot 100 per cent know what it is to be them any more than they can truly know what it is like to be us.

The ignorant saboteur can have different levels of sabotage – from the highly critical and demeaning kind who provoke all sorts of emotional responses in you, to the sympathetic kind who just do not understand what it is like to have such an inability to resist food, which of course can be very frustrating for you. This ignorance has the potential to disrupt your weight-loss effort nonetheless.

The Sceptic Saboteur

The sceptic saboteur is the type of person who, no matter what the evidence may say to the contrary, will permanently be sceptical towards you, which results in undermining anything you try to do, including losing weight. The sceptic is unlikely to offer any support and will try to take advantage of any information you may have given them to be sceptical about or use against you. All saboteurs have their own, often skewed, agendas, and making you feel bad about yourself is usually the sceptic's main tactic. If you are feeling bad about yourself, this makes them feel better about themselves, albeit only ever temporarily. Using the outright ploy of being sceptical and cynical about and towards you is a common one that you have to be aware of.

The Superior Saboteur

The superior type of saboteur is usually someone who has spent a lot of time and effort dieting and has successfully lost weight. They constantly compare your weight-loss efforts and approach to their own successful ones. This comparison is often presented and disguised as some kind of well-meaning help for you by learning from their own successful experiences. Yet with the superior type of saboteur, scratch the surface of their supposed help and you quickly find it is all about them and their own experiences of dieting. They will constantly go on about how much harder is was for them, why their reasons for being overweight are so much more important than yours. The superior type of saboteur will want the focus to be on them and any small amount of weight they may need to lose, which they always seem to have. They expect your emotional attentiveness and support, and there is nothing more irritating, and emotionally upsetting, as someone fretting about a small amount of weight, even if it is important to them, when you have still got a significant amount to lose. The superior saboteurs are always looking for an audience for their current weight-loss efforts and former achievement, but it will not do you any good to have to constantly attend to them and their need for emotional validation.

Also, the superior type of saboteur does not want you to succeed because the spotlight of success may move away from them. When someone has spent a lot of time and effort losing weight, quite often they enjoy the attention that comes with their success. They may perceive your dieting success as something that will take the attention away from them. The simplest way to avoid this is to stop you being successful by whatever means and encouraging your continued eating.

In the following part of this week's session you will meet Kate, Frank and Linda for one final time to help illustrate the types of saboteurs and assist you in identifying any potential saboteurs you may have in your life.

Case Study: Kate

'When I started to think about potential saboteurs, of course my sister Emma was not too far from my mind. I think that she's been sabotaging me in one form or another all my life. I particularly remember when I was at university and splitting up with my first boyfriend (who she'd been really jealous about). She rushed to

> visit me, loaded with boxes of chocolate, and sat there literally feeding them to me as she listened to my heartbreak. Of course I had no idea what she was up to, but I do remember noticing a sense of satisfaction in her when she left. I'd always assumed it was because my new boyfriend was out of the picture but Emma's always had such a skewed relationship with food she could have just as likely been satisfied at me consuming loads of chocolates when she didn't have one herself.
>
> 'If I get upset about things, my husband just wants to make it better for me. His idea of a quick fix is to bring me a box of chocolates, or a packet of shortbread biscuits, which he knows I really like. I know that he is only being thoughtful and kind, but sometimes I really do wish he wouldn't. He's one of those people who can eat anything and not gain an ounce, and he's really never been that fussed about food – if he's not interested in it he'll just leave it. So as sympathetic as he says he is to my overweight struggles, he just doesn't quite get it. But I have spoken to him about this, and now he tries to get me something else as a token of his love and concern – usually a bunch of flowers, which is lovely.

It may seem an emotionally upsetting concept to have to consider who in your life would either consciously (like Justine's feeder, or Kate's sister) or subconsciously (like Kate's husband) ruin your weight-loss plans, but they do, and most saboteurs are often very well known to you. You may not always be able to stop them tempting you with food, but knowing about them will give you back an important level of psychological control so you can decide when and what to eat.

Case Study: Frank

'When it comes to saboteurs I know that I'm probably my own worst enemy. If anything has upset me in the past, I've always kind of used it as an excuse to get a burger or kebab. I know through all the work and discoveries I've been making that, because I self-sabotage, I have to be the one to do something about it.

'Mum's had her own weight problems in the past, along with all the other things going on, and a few years ago started to go to a slimming club. She did okay and lost quite a bit of weight. But these days if there's any talk about weight loss for anyone – celebrities, family, members, neighbours, me – all she ever goes on about is her weight loss, "her journey". It's so annoying, but I have to try to not to take any notice, because if I do, I know it will end disastrously for me. I don't think she deliberately sets out to sabotage any of my efforts to lose weight, but she certainly doesn't help them in anyway by going on about her own. It's so ironic that she'll go on about her reasons for being overweight in the first place, the insecurities of her childhood (her dad died when she was a teenager) and just not see that she's done anything remotely similar to someone else.'

If you do not properly acknowledge and recognise sabotage, even if it is self-sabotaging like Frank, it will always have the potential to ruin even the most thought-out and determined weight-loss plans. Saboteurs will undermine your motivation to diet for any time in the future as well, more often than not without you knowing about it.

Case Study: Linda

'Both Rob and Dad have been so sceptical about many things in my life in the past. It is little wonder that when it comes to trying to lose weight they are going to be sceptical about that too. One minute Dad will take no notice of what I'm trying to do, then the next he'll ask me what I'm doing to lose weight. If I tell him anything he's dismissive about it or critical, saying I shouldn't have let myself go in the first place. Rob is not just sceptical and critical like Dad, he'll go out of his way to say something quite hurtful. For example, the other evening he said it was a wonder I could get so fat with my cooking abilities! When I got upset about it, he turned it around and made me feel guilty, saying I'd taken it the wrong way and I should lighten up. Then he laughed out loud because he'd said "lighten up" and me in the same sentence.

'Looking back to times when I have lost weight before, Rob definitely gets edgy about it. He'll say I looked fine as it was, which is so out of character for him I know something's up. Or he'll start being extra critical and nasty to me about anything and everything.

I remember once when I'd lost weight he went on and on about me buying the wrong kind of toilet cleaner – this from a man who's never once put the seat down on the toilet, let alone cleaned it. I think he sees it as a loss of his control over me if I'm doing something he doesn't want me to do, like losing weight. I'd never really considered it before, and it does really give me something to think about and be aware of. Not just with Rob, but with Dad too, because they both have their set agendas for me, which are to keep me near and doing things for them, regardless of whether I am happy doing it, fat or thin. I guess Rob thinks that if I'm fat it's more likely I'll stay.'

All saboteurs see your diet efforts as a threat to them for one reason or another, such as taking the attention away from them or, if you lose weight, they feel you may become more attractive to others and may ultimately leave them. Perhaps they do not want to be like Justine's feeder, left being the *'fat one'*. Or it could be, and this does happen more frequently than people credit, like Linda's partner, they are just not very nice people and take pleasure from the control of sabotaging others. You need to be aware of them to do something about them. Remember, saboteurs have a sense of their own inadequacies and their fragile sense of self, albeit subconciously in some cases, and will do anything to protect it.

Apart from the ignorant type of saboteur like Kate's husband, there is little you can do to change a saboteur's attitude and the way they think about and behave towards you. However, crucially, you can change your attitude towards *them* and you can predict their actions so you will be ready for them. Often the saboteur's best weapon is surprise: the surprise cake, the surprise change of mood towards you, the surprise change of plans. Doing something to take away that element of surprise will be to your psychological advantage and subsequent weight- loss benefit. Saboteurs may be like Justine's office feeder, blatantly bringing in cakes, or they may be the subtle, constantly undermining types, complimentary about you one moment then hurtful in the next. There are even types of saboteurs who will put extra sugars in your coffee, give you unrequested extra helpings of food or fill up your glass. Diet saboteurs do exist in all sorts of guises, so just being aware of them and vigilant to their tactics will give you and your diet a really strong advantage.

Saboteur Tips

One of the most important tips for you as the target of a saboteur is to understand about them and be ready for them, even if you do not know the specific actions and tactics they may take. Diet saboteurs can be relentless, so having a few tactics of your own will help you to deal with them.

Another tip to stop or manage any saboteurs in your life is to talk to them, if you feel they will listen. This often works best with the type of saboteur who is just ignorant of what it is like to struggle with your weight and does not understand why having a fridge full of cheesecakes and cream éclairs is unhelpful. You can talk to them in a nice way without going over the top, because often they just need a bit of education in the area of being a Take It type of eater. Also you can tell them this is not going to be forever, and that it is fine for them to have what they want, just as long as they do not leave all the tempting food around.

If the saboteur does continue to tempt you, tell them that you are trying to eat healthily and that for the time being you'd rather they didn't offer you anything. Keep some healthy snacks around to show that you mean business.

You could try to let the saboteur know directly that you are not eating what they bring in for you – say it like you mean it with no ambiguity or wavering. Be careful on this one, though, because some saboteurs enjoy the challenge of getting you to give in. Also watch out and be ready for the instant guilt trip they will send you on. Trying to make you feel like you are in the wrong for refusing or making a fuss about the food they have thought about, bought, and prepared just for you is a well-used saboteur ploy. If they really will not take no as an answer, take the piece of cake, the biscuits or whatever it is, tell them you will eat it later and either chuck it in the bin or give it to someone else who really wants it. Do not have it hanging around too long because the thought and temptation of it will probably prove too much, which is exactly what the saboteur wants.

Don't Get Paranoid

Do not start getting paranoid or obsessed by saboteurs – you just have to be ready for them. Other people will still bring in occasional things, like birthday cakes or Christmas treats. Use the tools you have learnt from *Stop Overeating* to resist and politely decline. You probably already know the type of person in your work, social or family life who feels better about themselves at the expense of your diet and psychological welfare.

When looking at people who sabotage your weight-loss intentions, I would not be really covering the topic of saboteurs if I did not take a brief look at the area of self-sabotage. This is where you deliberately and usually consciously put yourself in a position of temptation or emotional distress with the express intention of eating something that is not good for your weight loss. I do not want to spend too long on this topic, but want to emphasise that you need to be honest and aware of your thoughts and emotions when you know this is either happening or is likely to.

If you feel that you are self-sabotaging at any point because of an emotionally upsetting or distressing event, do an Backward Step analysis on it, find out what is going on for you emotionally and then employ and use the Mini Moment Intervention to stop yourself. If you feel further psychological exploration is required, analyse the events and people that cause you to self-sabotage by doing a Maxi Effect Analysis.

There will be times of huge emotional stresses in

everyone's lives, but what is important is not to add to the upset by using these times as an excuse to engage in any self-sabotaging behaviour and end up eating. It is just like dealing and coping with the other saboteurs in your life, so be honest and aware of your own emotions, thoughts, behaviours and – really importantly – your motivations. Remember you are always going to be your own best advocate and supporter when it comes to losing weight. With the right approach to saboteurs you can succeed.

Part 2
FOMO – The Fear of Missing Out

As you are reaching the end of your sessions, in the second part of this last session I want to briefly cover what is known as FOMO, which stands for the Fear Of Missing Out. This is that intense panicky sense and overwhelming anxiety you experience when the type of food you want to eat is being denied, not always but usually by yourself.

> ### Case Study: Helena
> *'I work as a ward nurse and often patients will give us boxes of chocolates as a thank you. It is so nice but does make my heart sink, because I know that after we've all had some chocolates, when it gets down to the ones that no one likes, I will always end up eating them. I don't even really like them myself, but I just have to have them if they are there. It's so frustrating because it's just wasted calories.'*

Helena is describing a typical fear of missing out, or FOMO, incident – a situation where food is being directly or indirectly offered to you in some way or another. It might be food you do not normally eat or particularly enjoy the taste of, like Helena and the chocolates she cannot resist. The fear of missing out has seen many diets end prematurely and is a really difficult concept for emotional eaters to both understand and overcome. On the one hand you know that the high-calorie and fattening food you are declining will not suddenly become permanently unavailable to you. The pastries and cakes will still be in the shops, the biscuits at work will still be there and, for Helena, the boxes of chocolates are still likely to be given by grateful patients. But on the other hand there is something inside you that overrides that logic and the need to have the food immediately is incredibly strong. In that split second, when the food is either being offered to you or you know it is there, it suddenly becomes impossible to resist and you just have to eat it.

There are many things which drive that urge, including the neurological motivation you looked at in the second session – Me and Food, What Happened? – when certain neurological receptors have been stimulated by the smell, sight or some strong association with a particular food and are demanding to be satisfied. Your whole relationship with food is also being tested at that precise moment, as are your beliefs about your ability to resist the food on offer. These, and all the other ideas and theories you have been exploring through the book, all play a part and contribute to that moment of panic and alarm, the FOMO moment, where the food you want is being denied or potentially taken away from you. It is already a highly complicated and intricate physical and emotional scenario before you even get to the part where you say either yes or no to the food.

So where does the fear of missing out come from? Often the origin of these fears, like so many emotional eating issues, is based on what has happened to you in your formative experiences. That is, what you have learnt through your direct experiences of availability, or more accurately the unavailability, of significant and important things in your life. This could be material things like food or possessions such as housing, money or warmth. However, quite likely your fears are just as much, if not more, rooted in and based on the unavailability of significant people in your life and not having the availability of emotional security. In Session One, Understanding the Emotional Chain of Events, you examined the importance of security and the subsequent impact that childhood insecurity can have on any of your relationships including a dysfunctional relationship with food.

Social Eating

If you have experienced a fear of missing out you know it can come at any time and in all shapes and sizes. However, social situations are particularly testing, because not only are you likely to miss out on the food on offer, but you may feel you are also missing out and excluding yourself from the social situation or interaction itself. Quite often social events are arranged around food (meeting friends for a meal, a barbecue, a lunchtime get-together, a dinner party) and the increase of all-you-can-eat restaurants is just an extra struggle emotional eaters could really do without. When you are dieting it can be a real dilemma both emotionally and socially. Do you not go with your friends? Or go and not eat? Or have something small?

Social settings can be a real problem for so many dieters anyway, but add in any emotional attachment to food, and the fear of missing out on it, and it becomes a complete headache. Then also add the 'not wanting to appear to make a fuss' or the possible issues and annoyances with bill splitting because you only had a starter, and a simple invitation to a meal can become a real predicament for anyone trying to stick to a diet and lose weight. The world, including your friends and family and their socialising, is going to continue, so you are going to have to find ways of adapting to it while dieting so you can carry on having fun with them.

During the previous sessions you have followed the examples of Kate, Frank and Linda. Although all of them had a level of childhood insecurity, Frank's case demonstrates how his mother's lack of attention, interest and care, and his insecurity about what was going to happen to him, was a major influence on him and has resulted in his emotional eating. In Frank's case, and for many others, the food itself was always available to him, too much so. Food became his emotional compensation for the lack of any real emotional availability or stability. So whenever he is faced with a situation where he has to deny himself something that he has such a strong emotional association with, it creates a huge psychological dilemma, an internal conflict which can override any logical thought. On the one hand Frank knows some foods do him no good, but on the other hand food has been such a comfort, a companion and source of pleasure for him that he finds it very hard to decline it.

Fear of missing out on food is going to be a challenge for any emotional eater, however you can help yourself when you feel that panic and fear trying to influence your actions and behaviours. You can quickly do a Mini Moment Intervention so you give yourself a crucial few minutes for the anxiety and fear to go and to lessen in intensity. Or you can do some Acknowledgement work, such as telling yourself that, although it is not fair that you are a Take It, not a Leave It, type of person when it comes to food, you are one and you need to acknowledge that. Anything at all which gets the plate of offered biscuits beyond your reach both physically and mentally will be crucial for you.

Planning Ahead

If you know that you have a social event coming up where food is likely to be an issue, like a family barbecue or dinner party, think in advance about what you can do to help yourself. Maybe half fill up with diet-friendly food before you go so hunger will not be influencing you as much. Remember, it is harder to make rational decisions about eating when you are genuinely hungry. Do not think that you are the only person experiencing something similar, because for all sorts of reasons – embarrassment, shame, not wanting to make a fuss – other people there are undergoing exactly the same dilemmas, however their fears may not always be related to food. You can still join in with the social situation and the food on offer, but you do not then have to have enormous amounts.

If you are going out for a meal, make sure you have something diet-friendly to bring with you. It does not have to be a massive amount of food, just something discreet that you know you can eat if you get hungry. Often just knowing you have a diet-friendly alternative, even without eating it, can be a good psychological tool to use because you can refuse certain foods or huge amounts of them knowing you have an alternative. If you are out for a meal at someone's house you can always have your snacks on the way home in the car – your host need never know. It may seem a waste of money especially if you are out for a meal in a restaurant with friends, but if you want to lose weight and be a successful dieter you are going to have to find a balance between being social and not ruining your diet. You want to be losing weight not friends!

In order to overcome your fears of missing out you need to adopt a completely different attitude and mindset. Instead of concentrating on what you are missing out on, you need to focus on what you gain from not eating the weight-increasing foods, such as the sense of achievement and satisfaction from not eating unnecessary calories and adding to your weight.

It is not a lot of fun being on a diet. They can be boring and hard, but it is also no fun at all being overweight and feeling that you blow your diet every few days because you believe you can't say no to food. You can, you just need to have alternatives, practices and a belief in yourself that for the duration of your diet you do not need to feel that you are missing out if you say no to temptation.

Part 3
Allowance Days

Add the FOMO to the saboteurs you looked at in the first part of this week's session and all the other emotional eating issues you have been examining in *Stop Overeating* and it is little wonder that sometimes you have ended up experiencing **allowance days**. These are the type of days that emotional eaters are so familiar with, the ones where something, anything, big or small, goes wrong and you end up eating because of it. You then quickly adopt the attitude and mindset that the diet has already failed for that particular day, so you allow yourself to eat anything at all. This could be food which you neither considered nor really wanted, but because of the diet having been ruined for that day you carry on eating. At its worst you then actively seek and buy food you have been avoiding because it has suddenly become allowed for that day.

If allowance days are not enough of a problem on their own, they do have a frequent habit of turning into allowance weeks and even allowance months. As you know, the longer it goes on, the harder it is to properly diet and lose weight.

Case Study: Tom

'It's so annoying. I'll be doing so well with the diet – I'll be sticking to it, eating sensibly, going to the gym and

will be losing weight. But then something will happen, it could be anything at all, that just ruins all my good intentions and saps my motivation and that's it for the rest of the day. Before I know it I'll be raiding the cupboards for all the fattening things I've hidden away, ordering takeaways, going to shops for food that I don't even like. And because I feel that I've blown it I might as well carry on.'

Maybe, like Tom, when you have an allowance day you feel that it is your fault you have given up, so you punish yourself for your failing with food. All emotional eaters promise and make deals with themselves that when they have an allowance day, they will start again the following day, or week. Failure to meet that promise becomes enough by itself to become an emotional trigger for an allowance day, week or month to continue.

Stay Focused

A good psychological tip to stop allowance days is to focus on what you can have to eat rather than what you cannot, because once you start even thinking about what you should not be having, those thoughts and images are going to be so much more difficult to do anything about. It is the 'do not think about a pink elephant' syndrome: the moment you try not to think about one you cannot stop yourself. Another tip is to mentally take yourself to a few moments in the future and think about how you would feel about yourself if you did blow the whole day.

Use the techniques you have learnt from the Mini Moment Intervention and give yourself a mindful and thoughtful 10 minutes.

Life is going to happen and things are going to upset you so unless you can lock yourself away in a stress- and emotion-free box for the duration of your weight loss, you are going to have to learn to cope with whatever comes your way without harming your diet or psychologically damaging yourself. It is at these points of hassle and provoked emotions that you need to make sure you apply what you have been learning in *Stop Overeating*: the complete understanding of the emotional chain of events in Session One, your relationships and beliefs about being an emotional eater explored in Session Two, and the psychological interventions – the Mini Moment Intervention, the Maxi Effect Analysis and the Challenge techniques – which you learnt in Session Three. Do one, a few or all of them to get you through that moment, but do not do nothing.

You are going to have moments, days and hours when, for one reason or another, the diet gets put on the back burner. But here is your choice: let it stay there on the back burner and let your commitment to losing weight eventually fizzle out. Or do something about it, with all the psychological tools you have been learning and applying.

No one said that it was going to be easy, but with the right psychological motivation and the emotional help within these pages, you can succeed. Remember, you are your own best advocate and champion. Through reading this book you have built a better awareness of yourself, making it easier to beat your emotional eating. In the next section, you'll learn more about the best foods to eat to complement all the work you've been doing.

28-day eating plan

When you undertake the *Stop Overeating* 28-day Eating Plan it's just as well to keep your psychological mind in gear. Try to remember all the good tips you have picked up from different diets in the past and apply them to this final one. Do not fall into the classic mind trap when it comes to the food – we have all done it – convincing yourself that because you are eating low-calorie, low-fat, 'good' foods you can have as much and as many of them as you like, which you know is not true. If you eat too much of just about anything – low-fat desserts, low-calorie drinks, reduced-fat meals or even fruit salad – you will stay overweight.

Getting Out of One Habit into Another

Lots of us have poor eating habits, constantly grazing and picking and never going for more than a few moments without eating something. As much as we may feel these little bits and pieces do not matter, your scales will tell you otherwise. Snacking in front of the TV is a classic time for all the good work you do during the day to be undone – you can eat so much food without even registering it. There is nothing wrong with a TV snack so long as it is a healthy one – *one* being the optimum word there. Also, one really good tip is to make the snack take as long as possible to eat: celery with a cottage cheese dip for example or half a dozen nuts in their shells. This is not just about the calories, it is about the time taken to eat. To satisfy your established grazing habits you almost have to trick yourself into believing that you are eating all the time, until you get into the habit of not doing so.

Fruit and Vegetables

Fruit and vegetables are key to taking control of your weight and health. Try to have at least one piece of fruit with each breakfast option; this can be either chopped up in something like cereal or porridge, or if you do not have time then a 200 ml (7 fl oz) glass of unsweetened fruit juice counts.

Fruit is great for weight loss as it consists mostly of water and can make the stomach feel full and stop cravings. It is also a good source of energy and nutrition. However, it should be eaten in moderation. Too much of anything, including virtuous fruit, will keep the weight on, so no huge fruit salads!

Fruit list, including portion size
- Apple, one whole
- Apricots, two medium

- Banana, one small
- Blackberries, handful
- Grapefruit, half fresh or one third of a can in fruit juice
- Grapes, handful
- Kiwi, one whole
- Mango, half fresh
- Melon, medium wedge
- Nectarine, one medium
- Orange, one medium
- Peach, one medium
- Pear, one whole
- Pineapple chunks in juice, 5–6 chunks
- Plums, three medium
- Raspberries, handful
- Satsumas, two medium
- Strawberries, handful

When it comes to the veggies you have with your meals, ideally you are looking to fill between one third and one half of your plate with vegetables. Starchy ones like potatoes, yams or sweet potatoes should be in moderation, and remember to not put extra butter on them. Also don't put any high-fat dressings on salads – see my recipes for low-fat salad dressings on page 260.

It can be helpful to think of vegetables in terms of colour. If there is no colour on your plate, think what vegetables can go on there to make it more colourful. Even when you are not on a diet, which if you follow *Stop Overeating* will happen, keep your vegetable portions high, because it is an easy way to maintain your weight loss.

Vegetable list, including portion size

- Asparagus, five spears
- Beans (French, broad, fine), four heaped tablespoons
- Broccoli, two spears
- Cabbage, two handfuls sliced
- Carrots, three heaped tablespoons
- Cauliflower, eight florets
- Celery, three sticks
- Chard, four heaped tablespoons
- Courgette, half large
- Kale, four heaped tablespoons
- Leek, one
- Lettuce, one bowlful
- Mushrooms, three to four heaped tablespoons
- Onions, one medium
- Parsnip, one large
- Peas (sugarsnap, garden, mangetout), three heaped tablespoons
- Peppers, half one
- Potatoes, one medium or four or five new
- Shallots, two to three
- Spinach, four heaped tablespoons
- Spring onions, eight onions
- Swede, three heaped tablespoons
- Sweetcorn, three heaped tablespoons
- Sweet potato, one medium
- Tomatoes, one medium or seven cherry
- Yams, three heaped tablespoons

How to Use the 28-day Eating Plan

I have designed this eating plan to ensure steady and sustainable weight loss with a variety of appetising and flavour-packed meals. There is nothing gimmicky or expensive about the plan. It is a straightforward programme of planned meals for you to follow while you undertake the psychological side of *Stop Overeating*. To make it as easy as possible, which is what we all need when losing weight, all the ingredients are fairly straightforward to find and are available from most major retailers. Also, I have designed these meals to be fairly quick to prepare, because, however much you may love cooking, when you are on a dedicated plan to lose weight, it is probably not the best idea to be in the kitchen for too long.

If you have to get meals ready for other family members, they can have what you are having – these meals are suitable for most people. Many former clients have found that giving other family members their meals was a practical option that worked well. If needed, they can be prepared fairly easily in tandem with the other meals you may have to prepare.

It is worth emphasising at this point that however tempting it may be to think it is too much effort to prepare different meals, remember why you are undertaking the whole *Stop Overeating* programme. Remind yourself that you are worth the effort of preparing special meals. Focus on moving forward and taking control of your emotional eating once and for all. Following the 28-day Eating Plan is going to be a key part of turning your life around.

When you begin a diet, it is common to look for fast weight-loss results, but a steady and continual weight loss will be much more attainable and sustainable. If you do a starvation diet, the psychological state of mind caused by acute hunger is in itself a cause of all types of emotions, which will more than likely lead to greater emotional eating in the long term. With this 28-day Eating Plan, you can lose weight in a practical and achievable way.

The eating plan consists of three healthy and filling meals each day, including a dessert after dinner. You can also eat two to three small snacks each day to keep you going between meals if you are tempted to pick up something unhealthy. You know yourself best – do you prefer to follow a strict diet with a planned variety of meals each day, or are you a more spontaneous person who likes to decide what you are going to eat each morning, depending on your daily routine? The eating plan is designed to work for you either way – you can follow each day as it is written or swap breakfasts, lunches and dinners around to fit in with what you are doing and what you like to eat. The best and most successful eating plan is the one that you will stick to – so decide how you are going to make the eating plan a success for you.

Supplement your breakfasts with fruit and your lunches and dinners with salads and unbuttered vegetables to fill your plate and keep you full for longer. Be careful of extra calories in your diet through drinks and sugars and be careful to limit your treats carefully. Where possible, use only skimmed milk for your cereal and in your tea and coffee. Do not add any extra sugar to your meals – a small teaspoon of clear honey will work just as well for sweetening if necessary. If you do have to use sugar, half a teaspoon goes a long way over cereal. Put the milk on first so the sugar does not sink to the bottom, leaving you wanting more. Porridge should be made with water not milk, and toast should be unbuttered.

The easy-to-follow recipes for each cooked or prepared meal (indicated in bold type in the eating plan) are at the end of the 28-Day Eating Plan, along with some suggested healthy and low-fat salad dressings.

Week 1

Day 1

Breakfast: Porridge (made with 40g/1½ oz oats and water) with cinnamon and a handful of raisins

Lunch: One crusty roll with one poached egg and one grilled sliced tomato

Dinner: **Tagliolini with almond pesto** (page 202)

Dessert: **Spiced orange sorbet** (page 251)

Day 2

Breakfast: One toasted plain bagel filled with one tablespoon of soft cheese

Lunch: **Carrot and coriander soup with homemade croutons** (page 244)

Dinner: **Mushroom and thyme risotto** (page 203)

Dessert: One-quarter of a small shop-bought flan case filled with fruit, served with one tablespoon of single cream

Day 3

Breakfast: Two slices of medium wholemeal bread filled with one grilled vegetarian sausage, sliced into four strips, and one grilled sliced tomato

Lunch: One jacket potato (no butter) with two tablespoons of tuna (canned in water or brine, drained) and chopped cucumber

Dinner: **Fish and rustic chunky chips** (page 204)

Dessert: Bought meringue nest, one tablespoon of fromage fraîs with grated dark chocolate topping

Day 4

Breakfast: One medium slice of wholemeal toast, one scrambled egg and one medium grilled tomato

Lunch: Homemade pasta salad: 100 g (4 oz) dried pasta cooked with selection of vegetables and one tablespoon of dressing

Dinner: **Blue cheese polenta with sun-dried peppers and mushrooms** (page 206)

Dessert: One piece of fresh fruit

Day 5

Breakfast: 40 g (1½ oz) Corn flakes with skimmed milk

Lunch: Cheese and tomato on two slices of medium toast

Dinner: **Winter vegetable casserole with herb dumplings** (page 208)

Dessert: Small pot of yoghurt

Day 6

Breakfast: Four fruit salad: pick four fruits from the fruit list (make sure anything canned is in a natural juice), add small amount of orange juice and one tablespoon of natural yoghurt

Lunch: One medium jacket potato with two tablespoons of cottage cheese, topped with paprika

Dinner: **Chicken stir-fry** (page 210)

Dessert: Two shop-bought Scotch pancakes, toasted with one teaspoon honey of and one tablespoon of fromage fraîs

Day 7

Breakfast: One grilled sausage, one grilled rasher lean bacon, one grilled tomato, four poached mushrooms and one poached egg

Lunch: One toasted wholemeal pitta cut into fingers with two tablespoons of houmous

Dinner: **Spinach base margherita pizza** (page 211)

Dessert: **Pineapple and ginger compote** (page 252)

Week 2

Day 8

Breakfast: Two Weetabix with skimmed milk

Lunch: **Butternut squash soup** (page 246), two crisp-breads with one tablespoon of cream cheese

Dinner: **Pasta twirls with kale and cheese** (page 213)

Dessert: **Chocolate soufflé** (page 253)

Day 9

Breakfast: Four fruit smoothie: any four fruits blended with a small pot of natural yoghurt

Lunch: One wrap with two tablespoons of cream cheese and salad

Dinner: **Spicy chicken with broccoli** (page 214)

Dessert: One third of a can of rice pudding, with one teaspoon of flaked almonds

Day 10

Breakfast: Two medium slices of wholemeal toast with one tablespoon of peanut butter between them

Lunch: One jacket sweet potato with one tablespoon of sour cream and chopped chives

Dinner: **Root vegetable curry** (page 215)

Dessert: One piece of fresh fruit

Day 11

Breakfast: One medium slice of wholemeal toast with 150 g (5 oz) baked beans

Lunch: Sliced vegetable crudités: celery, peppers,

carrots, cucumber, baby sweetcorn, with one pitta, toasted and cut into fingers, and two tablespoons of sour cream with chives

Dinner: **Grilled portobello mushrooms with Wensleydale cheese crumble** (page 217)

Dessert: Bought meringue nest with a handful of mixed berries and one tablespoon of single cream

Day 12

Breakfast: 40 g (1½ oz) reduced-sugar muesli mixed with one small pot of natural yoghurt

Lunch: Cheese and celery or chives toastie (no spreads or butter)

Dinner: **Creamy light macaroni cheese with butternut squash** (page 219)

Dessert: **Strawberry, vanilla and cherry compote** (page 254)

Day 13

Breakfast: Half a fresh grapefruit (or one third canned in natural juice, which can be used as one of the glasses of breakfast fruit juice), one medium slice of wholemeal toast with one tablespoon of cream cheese and Marmite

Lunch: A small cheese scone with a walnut, celery and apple salad

Dinner: **Stuffed cheesy peppers** (page 221)

Dessert: Small pot of yoghurt

Day 14

Breakfast: One grilled sausage, one grilled rasher lean bacon, one grilled tomato, four poached mushrooms and one poached egg

Lunch: One crusty roll with thin-sliced cheese and salad

Dinner: **Pan-fried pork chops and homemade apple sauce** (page 223)

Dessert: **Chocolate and ginger peaches** (page 255)

Week 3

Day 15

Breakfast: One scrambled egg on one slice of medium wholemeal toast, plus one slice of medium wholemeal toast (unbuttered) with one teaspoon of either jam, honey or marmalade

Lunch: **Broccoli and yellow pepper soup** (page 247), one middle slice of soda bread or two end slices

Dinner: **Pasta with sun-dried tomato pesto and feta cheese** (page 225)

Dessert: One piece of fresh fruit

Day 16

Breakfast: 40 g (1½ oz) Bran Flakes with skimmed milk

Lunch: Lean ham and tomato toastie (no butter)

Dinner: **Spicy root and lentil casserole** (page 226)

Dessert: **Mango and berry compote** (page 256)

Day 17

Breakfast: One raisin bagel toasted with two tablespoons
of cream cheese

Lunch: One medium jacket potato (no butter) with
150 g (5 oz) baked beans

Dinner: **Paprika chicken with asparagus** (page 227)

Dessert: One quarter of a small shop-bought flan case
filled with fruit, served with one tablespoon of
single cream

Day 18

Breakfast: Porridge (made with 40 g / 1½ oz oats and
water) with one teaspoon of flaked almonds

Lunch: One wrap with two tablespoons of soft cheese,
one tablespoon of sweetcorn, four chopped
pineapple chunks and rocket

Dinner: **Polenta with sautéed mushroom, courgettes
and goat's cheese** (page 228)

Dessert: **Berry ice-cream yoghurt with flaked
almonds** (page 257)

Day 19

Breakfast: 40 g (1½ oz) Rice Krispies with skimmed milk

Lunch: **Parsnip and apple soup** (page 249), crusty roll
(no butter)

Dinner: **Creamy salmon and broccoli pasta** (page 230)

Dessert: Bought meringue nest with one small chopped
banana and grated dark chocolate

Day 20

Breakfast: Porridge (made with 40 g / 1½ oz oats and water) with handful mixed berries

Lunch: One jacket sweet potato with one tablespoon of cream cheese, chopped red pepper and one tablespoon of houmous

Dinner: **Zesty yoghurt Greek lamb chops with aubergine and courgette grills** (page 231)

Dessert: Small pot of yoghurt

Day 21

Breakfast: One grilled sausage, one grilled rasher lean bacon, one grilled tomato, four poached mushrooms and one poached egg

Lunch: 150g (5 oz) baked beans on two slices of medium wholemeal toast (no butter)

Dinner: **Salmon spinach with spiced crème fraîche** (page 232)

Dessert: Two shop-bought Scotch pancakes, toasted with lemon juice and one teaspoon of honey

Week 4

Day 22

Breakfast: Two Oatibix with skimmed milk

Lunch: **Chilli, lentil and tomato soup** (page 250), with one slice medium wholemeal bread (no butter or spread)

Dinner: **Creamy mushroom spaghetti** (page 233)

Dessert: One piece of fresh fruit

Day 23

Breakfast: Banana smoothie: blend 1 small banana with 150 ml (¼ pt) skimmed milk

Lunch: One wholemeal pitta toasted and cut into fingers, with two tablespoons of cottage cheese topped with paprika

Dinner: **Chilli steaks and salsa** (page 235)

Dessert: **Apricot and walnut compote** (page 258)

Day 24

Breakfast: One medium slice of wholemeal toast, with one poached egg and one medium grilled tomato

Lunch: One jacket sweet potato with one teaspoon of sour cream and chopped chives

Dinner: **Warm gemelli with cherry tomato and artichoke salad** (page 236)

Dessert: One third of a can of rice pudding, with one tablespoon of chopped dates

Day 25

Breakfast: 50 g (2 oz) malted wheat cereal with skimmed milk

Lunch: One jacket sweet potato, two tablespoons of cottage cheese, topped with one tablespoon of sweetcorn

Dinner: **Chickpea curry with brown rice** (page 237)

Dessert: **Apple and pear meringue** (page 259)

Day 26

Breakfast: Porridge (made with 40g / 1½ oz oats and water) with one tablespoon of dried fruit mix

Lunch: One wrap with two tablespoons of houmous, one slice of lean ham and salad

Dinner: **Rocket pizza with poached egg** (page 238)

Dessert: Banana split: one small banana with two tablespoons of fromage fraîs and one tablespoon of chopped dates

Day 27

Breakfast: One reduced-fat croissant with half a tablespoon of soft cheese

Lunch: One wholemeal roll with one sliced grilled sausage and one teaspoon of mustard

Dinner: **Blue cheese omelette with rustic chunky chips** (page 239)

Dessert: Small pot of yoghurt

Day 28

Breakfast: One grilled sausage, one rasher lean bacon grilled, one grilled tomato, four poached mushrooms and one poached egg

Lunch: One jacket potato with one tablespoon of cream cheese, four or five chopped pineapple chunks and salad

Dinner: **Three-bean chilli and rice** (page 241)

Dessert: Bought meringue nest with two tablespoons of
             Greek yoghurt and a handful of pistachio nuts

Snacks

Healthy snacks are a must-have in any weight-loss plan,
but remember your two Qs: it is both about the quantity
and the quality. The quantity of any snack has to be in
moderation – so no eating half packets of rice cakes in one
go. Also, and just as importantly, it is going to be about
the quality of your snack, it needs to be low-calorie – no
bars of chocolate just because they are small. Two to three
snacks a day would be reasonable, and make sure you vary
them – you do not want to get to the end of the day having
eaten three bags of crisps, no matter how low in fat and
calories they are. When you have time, try to make the
snacks last and acknowledge them. I am not saying you
have to form a long-lasting relationship with them, but do
not simply cram them down. If you do, all you are doing
is getting ready for the next eating opportunity, which may
not be so good for you if a planned meal is too far away.
A small handful of nuts in shells is good because removing
the shells will take some time. In situations like these it is
about tricking the eating habits – this is about using time,
not calories. Try to make a note of what times of the day
you snack; is it usually in front of the TV, or when you
are at work? It is okay to have specific times to take a few
moments to yourself, but you are going to need to keep the

calorie intake to a bare minimum.

Do not fall in to the classic dieter's trap of rewarding your hard work sticking to your eating plan during the day by negating some of the hard work at the end of the day. It is just all too easy to want to reward your virtuous eating, but you know what will happen – one day's reward will lead to another day, as one chocolate digestive will lead to another, so be aware of what you are eating all the time.

If you want to acknowledge and mark your eating plan achievements, there is absolutely nothing wrong with that. There are lots of things you can do which do not involve eating. Why not research something for pleasure on the internet, read a book or magazine, do some personal pampering. Anything at all for a few minutes, just to remind yourself what you are doing, who you are doing it for and how well you are doing. It is important because by acknowledging your achievements, no matter how small, it will help to keep you motivated and lose weight. If you get a bit stuck or self-conscious about allowing yourself these few moments, then remind yourself of a few of the reasons why you are undertaking the *Stop Overeating* plan, such as wanting to lose weight, develop a healthy relationship with food and, of course, stop your emotional eating once and for all.

Here is a list of just a few low-calorie, low-fat snacks. There are plenty out there and it would be good for you to research some others. This will be psychologically beneficial to you because you are being active about your weight loss and taking control of your eating.

- One portion of fresh fruit
- Handful of dried fruit
- Small handful of nuts
- Two dried figs
- Celery sticks with one tablespoon of cottage cheese
- Two breadsticks with one tablespoon of houmous
- One hard-boiled egg
- Two microwaved poppadums with one tablespoon mint and yoghurt
- Two rice cakes with Marmite
- Two Jaffa cakes
- Four squares of dark chocolate
- 25 g (1 oz) Twiglets
- One medium packet of Quavers/French Fries/ Wotsits
- Small bag (11 g / ½ oz) of salted/plain popcorn

A couple of practical notes: all the oven temperatures are based on a fan oven, so increase the temperature accordingly for a non-fan oven. I have used dried herbs for all the recipes, but you can use fresh chopped ones if you prefer. All the recipes serve two, unless otherwise stated.

Dinner Recipes

Day 1: Tagliolini with Almond Pesto

A different twist for any pasta and pesto lovers. This is a really tasty and satisfying dish to kick-start your weight loss.

Ingredients

50 g (2 oz) basil
1 tbsp ground almonds
30 g (1 oz) Parmesan cheese, finely grated (you can use any hard cheese)
Pinch of ground sea salt
Pinch of freshly ground black pepper
250 g (9 oz) fresh tagliolini
Splash of skimmed milk (optional)

Method

1. With a food processor or hand blender mix together the basil, almonds, cheese, salt and pepper. Add a splash of skimmed milk if the mixture looks too dry.
2. Cook the pasta in unsalted boiling water according to packet instructions and make sure it is drained for at least 2 minutes.
3. Combine the pasta with the basil mixture in a large bowl. Sprinkle with a little extra Parmesan cheese if desired.

Day 2: Mushroom and Thyme Risotto

This is a delicious and deceptively simple meal. To add a little extra taste to the dish, you can substitute a small glass of white wine for some of the stock.

Ingredients

1 tsp olive oil
350 g (12 oz) mushrooms, sliced
½ tsp thyme
120 g (4½ oz) risotto rice
1 l (1¾ pt) hot vegetable stock
30 g (1 oz) Parmesan cheese, grated

Method

1. Heat the oil in a medium saucepan and sauté the mushrooms for 2–3 minutes, then turn down to a low heat and add the thyme and rice.
2. Add a quarter of the stock and keep the rice simmering, stirring continually. When the stock is absorbed add the next quarter of the stock, stirring continually again. Add the remaining stock gradually, making sure each addition is absorbed before adding the next. Simmer until the stock is all absorbed and the rice is cooked thoroughly.
3. Serve immediately with a sprinkle of grated cheese on top.

Day 3: Fish and Rustic Chunky Chips

There is no need to miss out on a firm favourite just because you are dieting. Other members of your family will love the chunky chips too – everyone does – so make sure you do a few extra for them.

Ingredients
2 medium potatoes, washed and unpeeled
1 tbsp vegetable oil
¼ tsp celery salt
2 x 150 g (5 oz) cod fillets
Juice of 1 lemon
Salt and freshly ground black pepper
1 large free-range egg
50 g (2 oz) Panko breadcrumbs, also known as Japanese breadcrumbs

Method
1. Preheat your oven to temperature 180°C/400°F/Gas 6.
2. Cook the rustic chips in one of these two ways:
   - Cut the potatoes into long chip shapes, rinse under a cold tap and pat dry. Toss the potato with a little oil and the celery salt and then spread on a non-stick baking tray. Roast for 35–45 minutes, turning them a quarter turn now and then, until golden brown and crisp all over.
   - Or cook the coated potatoes in the microwave until just underdone, then carefully cut them into long chip shapes and either grill or bake in the oven until golden brown.

3. For the fish, place the fillets in a bowl, sprinkle over the lemon juice and season well. Coat each cod fillet with beaten egg and then breadcrumbs. Place on a lightly oiled baking tray and put in the oven for 15–20 minutes. Once the fish is cooked turn the oven up to 200°C/425°F/Gas 7 to brown the chunky chips.

Day 4: Blue Cheese Polenta with Sun-dried Peppers and Mushrooms

Corn maize polenta is available from most supermarkets. It is a satisfying product, easy to cook, and you do not need too much of it to make you feel full. Here it is served with tasty blue cheese, mushrooms and peppers, but you can combine it with lots of different veggies and use a different cheese if you don't like blue.

Ingredients
1 tbsp vegetable oil
200 g (7 oz) mushrooms, any type, sliced
50 g (2 oz) sun-dried peppers, rinsed and sliced
1 garlic clove, crushed
½ tsp thyme
½ tsp parsley
Pinch of ground sea salt
Pinch of freshly ground black pepper
100 g (4 oz) dry, uncooked polenta
50 g (2 oz) Danish blue cheese

Method
1. Heat the oil in a griddle or frying pan. Sauté the mushrooms and peppers until tender with the garlic, herbs and seasoning.
2. While the mushrooms and peppers are cooking, make the polenta according to packet instructions with water and omit any butter if it is included in the cooking instructions.

3. Divide the polenta between two gratin dishes and top with the cooked mushrooms and peppers.

4. Sprinkle with crumbled cheese then place under a hot grill for 2–5 minutes, until the cheese melts. Serve with a spinach and rocket side salad with one of the salad dressing recipes at the end of the recipes.

Day 5: Winter Vegetable Casserole with Herb Dumplings

Dumplings are not the first thing you would think about when you are on a diet. This is a great recipe, which allows you to enjoy what, for many, is the essential part of any casserole.

Ingredients

1 garlic clove, minced
1 medium leek, chopped
1 medium sweet potato, peeled and diced
2 medium carrots, peeled and diced
2 medium parsnips, peeled and diced
275 ml (½ pt) vegetable stock
1 can (400 g/14 oz) chopped tomatoes
Pinch of ground sea salt
100 ml (4 fl oz) sour cream

Herb Dumplings

100 g (4 oz) plain flour
½ tsp baking powder
½ tsp mixed herbs
30 g (1 oz) low-fat spread, grated if possible
½ tsp mustard powder (optional)

Method

1. In a large pan, cook the garlic and vegetables with the stock, simmering for about 45 minutes until the vegetables are tender. Add the canned tomatoes, season to taste and bring back to a simmer.

2. While the vegetables are cooking, make the dumplings by combining the flour, baking powder, herbs, spread (and mustard powder, if using). Add a little water until the dumpling mix is tacky and not too dry.

3. Divide the mixture into four equal balls and place on top of the vegetable casserole. Do not stir them in, just allow them to sit on top. Cook for 8–10 minutes until the dumplings have just about doubled in size.

4. When cooked, stir the sour cream in to the casserole and serve straight away.

Day 6: Chicken Stir-fry

I love stir-fries – they are so quick, easy and a really tasty meal. They are also particularly good if you are pushed for time. This is a chicken recipe, but can easily be made using either tofu or vegetarian chicken-style chunks.

Ingredients

60 ml (2 fl oz) chicken stock
450 g (1 lb) skinless chicken breast fillet strips
1 tsp vegetable oil
¼ tbsp cayenne pepper
1 tsp ground ginger
110 g (4 oz) asparagus, sliced along length
1 medium red or yellow pepper, sliced
110 g (4 oz) mushrooms, sliced
1 medium carrot, cut into thin batons
2–3 spring onions, sliced along length
1 tsp soy sauce (optional)

Method

1. Heat the chicken stock in a non-stick wok or frying pan over a medium heat. Add the chicken strips and cook until almost done.
2. Heat the oil in the pan/wok and add the cayenne pepper, ginger, and vegetables for 1–3 minutes until any remaining liquid has evaporated away.
3. Cook until everything is tender, drain the excess stock and set the mixture aside in a bowl.
4. Serve immediately, with a little soy sauce, to taste, if you wish.

Day 7: Spinach Base Margherita Pizza (Makes one 25 cm / 10 in pizza)

When I have been on a diet, one of the biggest problems I have found is missing out on what others are eating. In my house, Saturday night is pizza night, so I developed this recipe specifically not to miss out on pizza. You can make and freeze the bases in advance too. The spinach base is delicious but have a knife and fork on standby to prevent too much mess!

Ingredients

Base:

100 g (4 oz) fresh spinach, finely chopped or roughly
   blended
1 large free-range egg
50 g (2 oz) mozzarella cheese, grated
1 tsp basil
½ tsp oregano
½ tsp paprika (optional)
25 g (1 oz) uncooked, dry polenta

Pizza Topping:

250 g (9 oz) passata
½ garlic clove, crushed
25g (1 oz) cheese, grated

Method

1. Set the oven temperature to 180°C/400°F/Gas 6.
2. For the base, blend together the fresh spinach, egg, grated

mozzarella, basil, oregano, paprika and dry polenta until they are as smooth as possible. Line a baking tray with either a silicone baking sheet or parchment paper (do not use greaseproof paper as it will stick). Spread the mixture on the baking sheet making a 25 cm (10 in) diameter base. Bake for 12–15 minutes or until the edges begin to brown. Allow to cool, then carefully remove the parchment paper.

3. For the pizza topping, mix the passata and garlic together, spread on the cooled base, leaving 1–2 cm (½–¾ in) around the outside, sprinkle the cheese and place in a hot oven at 200°C/425°F/Gas 7 or under a hot grill for 3–5 minutes, until the cheese melts.

4. Serve with a side salad. You can also add a few sliced onions, mushrooms or any veggies of your choice.

Day 8: Pasta Twirls with Kale and Cheese

Kale can be a bit overlooked, but like most green vegetables it is full of nutrients. Combined with some tangy cheese, it can be a surprising find for a lot of dieters and non-dieters alike.

Ingredients

250 g (9 oz) fresh fusilli pasta
1 tbsp olive oil
1 garlic clove, crushed
110 g (4 oz) kale, stalks removed, washed and chopped
Pinch of ground sea salt
Pinch of freshly ground black pepper
120 ml (4 fl oz) vegetable stock
200 g (7 oz) cannellini beans, rinsed and drained
20 g (¾ oz) Parmesan cheese, shaved
¼ small chilli, finely chopped (optional)

Method

1. Cook the pasta in plain boiling water according to packet instructions and then drain.
2. In a medium saucepan heat the oil then add the garlic, kale and seasoning. Cook for 1 minute or until the kale starts to wilt.
3. Add the stock, bring it all to the boil and simmer for 5 minutes or until the liquid is nearly evaporated.
4. Finally, add the pasta and cannellini beans and keep stirring until everything is hot.
5. Top with cheese and chopped chilli, if you wish.

Day 9: Spicy Chicken with Broccoli

This recipe adds a bit of a kick to the everyday, which is sometimes needed when you are on a diet. You can also make this meal with any vegetarian substitutes.

Ingredients
2 broccoli heads, cut into florets
1 tbsp vegetable oil
1 red chilli, deseeded and sliced
1 garlic clove, sliced
6–8 pitted black olives, rinsed
450 g (1 lb) pre-cooked skinless chicken breasts, cut into
    bite-sized pieces

Method
1. Steam the broccoli until tender.
2. Heat the oil in a large saucepan, then sauté the chilli and garlic for 1 minute. Add the broccoli, olives and chicken, and stir until warm.

Day 10: Root Vegetable Curry

I love a curry but they are not the first thing dieters consider eating as they are generally associated with lots of high-calorie creamy sauces and oils. However, you do not have to miss out. I have come up this great curry using a little bit of coconut powder, which is a great substitute for the high-calorie ingredients of traditionally cooked curries.

Ingredients

2 medium carrots, diced
2 medium parsnips, diced
1 medium sweet potato, diced
1 small celeriac, diced
240 ml (8 fl oz) vegetable stock
1 tsp curry powder
½ tsp thyme
Pinch of ground sea salt
Pinch of freshly ground black pepper
1 tbsp coconut powder, mixed with cold water to a paste
1 tbsp natural yoghurt
1 tbsp brown rice or a microwaved poppadum (optional)

Method

1. Cook the diced vegetables in water until tender and drain well.
2. Add the stock, curry powder, thyme and seasoning to the pan and simmer for 5 minutes, uncovered, to allow

some of the liquid to evaporate. Stir occasionally so there is no sticking when it is all cooked.

3. Add the coconut paste and cook for a further minute, stirring constantly. Remove from the heat and stir in the yoghurt just before serving.

4. Serve with either one tablespoon of plain brown rice or one microwaved poppadum. This is a substantial meal, so you may not need the rice.

Day 11: Grilled Portobello Mushrooms with Wensleydale Cheese Crumble

Mushrooms are a great dieter's friend, but I would be the first to admit they can sometimes be a little bit bland. Jazzing them up with just a small amount of tangy cheese is a great way of enjoying a filling amount of mushrooms. I have used Wensleydale cheese, but any crumbly cheese will do just as well.

Ingredients

½ tsp basil
Pinch of ground sea salt
Pinch of freshly ground black pepper
4 large portobello mushrooms, cleaned and stalks
    removed
2 medium tomatoes, cut into thick slices
1 garlic clove, crushed
1 tbsp olive oil
75 g (3 oz) Wensleydale cheese

Method

1. Sprinkle the basil, salt and pepper evenly over the mushrooms and sliced tomatoes.
2. Sauté the garlic in a hot, lightly oiled frying pan or griddle, then add the mushrooms and cook for 2–3 minutes or until tender, turning once (cook them upside down first so that when they are turned over the excess liquid can drain out).
3. Remove the mushrooms from the pan, then add the tomatoes to the pan and cook for 1 minute.

4. Place the tomatoes on top of the mushrooms, and crumble the Wensleydale cheese evenly over the top. Place under a hot grill until the cheese has melted.

5. Serve with a selection of two or three unbuttered vegetables from the vegetable list. The mushrooms go well with green beans, new potatoes and sweetcorn.

Day 12: Creamy Light Macaroni Cheese with Butternut Squash

A firm favourite made extra tasty with some delicious butternut squash. You can add a sprinkling of chilli powder or paprika before baking for a spicy flavour. Serves three to four.

Ingredients

*250 g (9 oz) butternut squash, peeled and cut in to 1-cm
  (½-in) cubes*
125 ml (4 fl oz) vegetable stock
60 ml (2 fl oz) skimmed milk
1 garlic clove, crushed
Pinch of ground sea salt
Pinch of freshly ground black pepper
1 tbsp Greek yoghurt
25 g (1 oz) Gruyère cheese, grated
15 g (½ oz) Parmesan cheese, grated
150 g (5 oz) uncooked whole-wheat macaroni
1 tbsp olive oil
50 g (2 oz) Panko breadcrumbs (Japanese breadcrumbs)
Sprinkle of chilli powder or paprika (optional)

Method

1. Preheat the oven to 180°C/400°F/Gas 6.
2. Combine the squash, stock, milk, garlic and seasoning in a medium saucepan and bring to the boil over a medium-high heat.

3. Reduce the heat and simmer until the squash is tender, then remove from the heat, allow to cool for 5 minutes and spoon into a blender along with half of the cooking liquid. Allow steam to escape for 2 minutes, then blend until smooth.

4. Stir in the Greek yoghurt and both cheeses, saving a little for the topping.

5. While the squash is cooking, cook the pasta according to packet instructions and drain.

6. Add the pasta to the squash mixture and stir together, then spread evenly into a deep ovenproof dish.

7. Finally, in a lightly oiled frying pan gently brown the breadcrumbs. Remove from the heat, stir in the remaining cheese and sprinkle evenly over the hot pasta mix. Top with the chilli powder or paprika, if using. Bake in the oven for 25 minutes or until bubbling.

Day 13: Stuffed Cheesy Peppers

It may be a blast from the past, but stuffed peppers are always a reliable, satisfying and tasty dinner. You can change the flavours easily by swapping the herbs used or adding garlic. I like the flavour of Edam but you could use any hard cheese.

Ingredients

2 medium peppers, any colour
200 g (7 oz) cooked brown rice
1 tsp dried basil
6–8 pitted olives, rinsed and chopped
Pinch of ground sea salt
Pinch of freshly ground black pepper
75 g (3 oz) Edam cheese, grated
1 tbsp olive oil

Method

1. Preheat the oven to 180°C/400°F/Gas 6.
2. Cut the top off the peppers and scoop out the core and seeds.
3. Mix the rice, basil, olives, seasoning, two-thirds of the cheese and the oil together. Pack the rice mixture into the peppers, replace the tops of the peppers and cook in a hot oven for 10–15 minutes.
4. When cooked, remove and discard the pepper tops (test that the peppers are tender at the top of the pepper: any further down and it may split). Sprinkle the remaining

cheese over the top and put back in the oven for 2 minutes until the cheese has melted.

5. Serve with a selection of two or three unbuttered vegetables from the vegetable list. The peppers go well with grilled mushrooms and courgettes.

Day 14: Pan-fried Pork Chops and Homemade Apple Sauce

Pork chops with apple sauce is a really great combination of traditional flavours and with a few vegetables this makes a satisfying and healthy dinner.

Ingredients

2 medium pork chops, fat removed
Pinch of ground sea salt
Pinch of freshly ground black pepper
50 g (2 oz) plain flour
1 tbsp vegetable oil
1 medium cooking apple or 2 firm eating apples
2 tsp caster sugar
1 tsp lemon juice (optional)

Method

1. Season the chops with the salt and pepper, then cover with the flour and cook in a medium oiled frying pan or griddle for 5–8 minutes, depending on thickness. Turn the chops once and cook them for a further 3–5 minutes or until they are completely cooked through.

2. While the chops are cooking, peel, core and chop the apple then cook in a small saucepan. Add the sugar and lemon juice, bring to the boil and simmer for 3–4 minutes, adding a tiny bit of water if the apples get a little sticky in the pan.

3. Once they are cooked, blend or mash the apples – the finer you can get them the better. Serve on the side with the pork.

4. Serve with a selection of two or three unbuttered vegetables from the vegetable list. A leek and potato mash complements the pork dish very well.

Day 15: Pasta with Sun-dried Tomato Pesto and Feta Cheese

A really delicious take on a pasta dinner, the sun-dried tomatoes are a great accompaniment to the pasta and the creamy feta adds just the right amount of taste balance.

Ingredients
250 g (9 oz) fresh linguine
110 g (4 oz) sun-dried tomatoes, drained if in oil
½ tsp basil
2 tbsp ground or flaked almonds
1 garlic clove, crushed
Pinch of ground sea salt
Pinch of freshly ground black pepper
20 g (¾ oz) Parmesan cheese
30 g (1 oz) feta cheese

Method
1. Cook the pasta according to packet instructions and drain through a sieve so you can retain 220 ml (7 fl oz) of its cooking water.
2. Return the pasta to the pan and cover to keep hot.
3. Finely chop or food-process the sun-dried tomatoes and add the basil, almonds, garlic, seasoning and Parmesan cheese. Combine the tomato mixture with half the saved pasta water, mix together and keep adding the water until you have the thickness you desire. Add the tomato mixture to the pasta and mix until the pasta is well coated.
4. Serve with the feta cheese crumbled over the top.

Day 16: Spicy Root and Lentil Casserole

A lovely satisfying warmer, which is not just for winter and is a handy meal that can be also be frozen for later. You can also add the dumplings from Day 5 if required.

Ingredients
1 tbsp vegetable oil
1 onion, chopped
1 garlic clove, crushed
1 medium potato, peeled and cut into chunks
3 carrots, peeled and thickly sliced
2 parsnips, peeled and thickly sliced
1 tbsp curry powder
1–1.5 l (1¾–2½ pt) vegetable stock
½ can (200 g/7 oz) green lentils
1 tbsp plain yoghurt or fromage fraîs

Method
1. Heat the oil in a large saucepan and sauté the onion and garlic.
2. Add the potatoes, carrots and parsnips and keep stirring for 3 minutes.
3. Add the curry powder and the stock, then bring the mixture to the boil.
4. Reduce the heat, add the lentils, cover and simmer for 15–20 minutes until the vegetables are tender and the sauce has thickened.
5. Stir in the plain yoghurt or fromage fraîs just before serving.

Day 17: Paprika Chicken with Asparagus

A nice quick meal that is high on taste and low on prep, we all need a few of these to help to keep us on the diet track. It is another good standby if you are short on time but need a proper meal to stop any snacking and picking later.

Ingredients

1 tbsp vegetable oil
1 tbsp paprika
4 skinless chicken breast fillets
300 g (11 oz) asparagus

Method

1. Mix the oil and paprika to a paste and rub all over the chicken breasts. Cook on a lightly oiled frying pan or griddle for 10–12 minutes until the chicken is becoming slightly charred and is cooked through when tested.
2. Halfway through cooking the chicken, add the asparagus to the griddle or frying pan and cook until it is tender.
3. Serve all together with a selection of two or three unbuttered vegetables from the vegetable list. Some sugarsnap peas and a sweet potato mash complement this meal nicely.

Day 18: Polenta with Sautéed Mushroom, Courgettes and Goat's Cheese

I have only recently discovered polenta and have to admit I'm a huge fan. I have suggested mushrooms, courgettes and goat's cheese, but this is a 'using things up in the fridge' recipe as polenta goes with just about everything.

Ingredients

1 tbsp vegetable oil
200 g (7 oz) mushrooms, any type, sliced
1 medium courgette, sliced
½ tsp thyme
½ tsp parsley
1 tsp crushed garlic
Pinch of ground sea salt
Pinch of freshly ground black pepper
110 g (4 oz) dry, uncooked polenta
30 g (1 oz) goat's cheese, sliced

Method

1. Heat the oil in frying pan or griddle and sauté the mushrooms and courgette until tender, then add the herbs, garlic and seasoning.
2. Cook the polenta according to packet instructions, omitting any butter.
3. Once cooked, divide the polenta between two gratin dishes and top with the mushrooms and courgette.
4. Place the sliced goat's cheese evenly over the top and

place under a hot grill for 2–5 minutes until the cheese bubbles and melts.

5. Serve with a spinach and rocket side salad with one of the salad dressing recipes at the end of the recipes.

Day 19: Creamy Salmon and Broccoli Pasta

Salmon and broccoli is a classic combination, and why not? It is a real diet-friendly one too – add a bit of pasta and you have an appetising and satisfying meal in no time at all.

Ingredients

75 g (3 oz) pasta shells, dried weight
2 broccoli heads, cut into florets
1 tbsp vegetable oil
1 leek, finely chopped
75 g (3 oz) garlic and herb cream cheese
6 tbsp semi-skimmed milk
150 g (5 oz) salmon fillets, cut into 2.5-cm (1-in)cubes
Pinch of ground sea salt
Pinch of freshly ground black pepper

Method

1. Cook the pasta according to packet instructions, then drain.
2. Steam the broccoli for 10 minutes and remove from the heat.
3. In a large saucepan, heat the oil and sauté the leek for 5 minutes. Stir in the cream cheese and milk, then add the salmon pieces and cook until they turn opaque (about 6–8 minutes).
4. Once everything is cooked, combine it together, season and serve straight away with side salad.

Day 20: Zesty Yoghurt Greek Lamb Chops with Aubergine and Courgette Grills

This is lovely Mediterranean take on an old favourite with some traditional Greek-style vegetables.

Ingredients

1 garlic clove, crushed

½ tsp thyme

1 lemon, zest and juice

4 lamb chops or cutlets, fat removed

1 tbsp olive oil

50 g (2 oz) Greek yoghurt

Pinch of ground sea salt

Pinch of freshly ground black pepper

1 medium aubergine, sliced

1 medium courgette, sliced

Method

1. Mix the garlic, thyme and lemon juice together and rub into the chops or cutlets. Then cook them in a lightly oiled frying pan or griddle for 5–7 minutes.
2. Mix the Greek yoghurt and lemon zest with seasoning.
3. Cover the chops on one side with the yoghurt mix and grill for a further 2 minutes.
4. Sauté the aubergine and courgette in a hot frying pan or griddle for 3–5 minutes.
5. Serve with new potatoes and baby carrots or any two or three unbuttered vegetables from the vegetable list.

Day 21: Salmon Spinach with Spiced Crème Fraîche

Another quick favourite, and having a spicy accompaniment which you can moderate to your own taste is a great way of enhancing this dinner.

Ingredients

1 tbsp vegetable oil
150 g (5 oz) skinless salmon fillet
250 g (9 oz) spinach, washed
2 lemon wedges
2 tbsp low-fat crème fraîche
½ tsp paprika (optional)

Method

1. Heat the oil in a frying pan or griddle and fry the salmon on each side for 6–8 minutes. At the same time, steam the spinach until it starts to wilt. Make sure it is well drained and add to the salmon for 2 minutes.
2. Serve with lemon wedges and gently heated crème fraîche, sprinkle with some paprika if required. Serve with either a dressed side salad or potato and swede mash.

Day 22: Creamy Mushroom Spaghetti

When you are on a weight-loss plan, sometimes socialising can go out of the window. This is a great recipe for having friends around for a meal. Add some garlic bread for them, not you, and they will not even know you are giving them a meal from your eating plan.

Ingredients

75 g (3 oz) spaghetti (dry weight)
1 tbsp vegetable oil
½ onion, finely chopped
350 g (12 oz) mushrooms, any type, chopped not
    too small
2 garlic cloves, crushed
Pinch of ground sea salt
Pinch of freshly ground black pepper
55 ml (2 fl oz) white wine
½ tsp thyme
55 ml (2 fl oz) single cream
15 g (½ oz) Parmesan cheese, grated
½ tsp parsley

Method

1. Cook the spaghetti according to packet instructions, drain and keep warm.
2. While the spaghetti is cooking, heat the oil in a large saucepan, add the onion, mushrooms, garlic and seasoning and sauté for 10 minutes or until mushrooms have browned.

3. Add the wine and thyme and cook for a further 2 minutes or until most of the liquid evaporates, stirring occasionally.

4. Remove the pan from the heat and add the cooked pasta, cream, Parmesan cheese and parsley, tossing to combine.

Day 23: Chilli Steaks and Salsa

A tasty meal for any day, but again this a good one for a meal with friends. The zingy homemade salsa is a great accompaniment too.

Ingredients

2 x 100 g (4 oz) 1 cm (½ in) thick steaks, excess fat removed
1 tsp chilli powder
2 pinches of ground sea salt
1 tbsp vegetable oil
2 tomatoes, diced
2 tsp lime juice
1 tsp coriander

Method

1. Sprinkle both sides of the steak with chilli powder and a pinch of salt, cook in a lightly oiled frying pan or griddle on a medium heat for 2–4 minutes per side for medium-rare.
2. Remove the steak from the pan or griddle and cover with foil to keep warm, leaving the remaining meat juice in the pan.
3. For the salsa, mix the tomatoes, lime juice, coriander and one pinch of salt in the pan the steak was cooked in.
4. Keep stirring until the tomatoes soften – about 3 minutes. Serve the steaks topped with the salsa and an undressed side salad.

Day 24: Warm Gemelli with Cherry Tomato and Artichoke Salad

Another lovely pasta meal. Artichokes can often be overlooked but they are a delicious vegetable that can be easily bought canned from most major retailers.

Ingredients
250 g (9 oz) fresh gemelli pasta
350 g (12 oz) asparagus, sliced
2 tbsp red wine vinegar
1 tbsp balsamic vinegar
1 tbsp olive oil
Pinch of ground black pepper
125 g (4½ oz) rocket
75 g (3 oz) cherry tomatoes, halved
200 g (7 oz) artichoke hearts, rinsed, drained and quartered

Method
1. Cook the pasta according to packet instructions. During the last 2 minutes of cooking time, add the asparagus to the pan and cook until tender, then drain.
2. While the pasta is cooking combine vinegars, oil and pepper in a large bowl, stirring vigorously with a whisk.
3. Add the cooked pasta mixture, rocket, tomatoes and artichokes and toss with the vinegar mix. Serve straight away.

Day 25: Chickpea Curry with Brown Rice

Brown rice is a real dieter's friend – it is great high-fibre, filling food, giving slow-release sugars and carbs, so it keeps you full and stops you snacking. Serves four.

Ingredients

1 tbsp vegetable oil
1 large onion, diced
½ tsp garam masala
1 can (400 g/14 oz) chickpeas, rinsed and drained
1 can (400 g/14 oz) chopped tomatoes, half drained of
 its juice
½ tsp ground coriander
175 g (6 oz) baby spinach (can use frozen, but you may
 need to drain the excess fluid off)
1½ tbsp coconut powder, mixed to paste with cold water
Pinch of ground sea salt
150 g (5 oz) cooked brown rice

Method

1. Heat the oil in a medium saucepan, add the onion and sauté for 5 minutes or until it is tender.
2. Stir in the garam masala and cook for 30 seconds, stirring constantly.
3. Add the chickpeas, tomatoes, coriander and spinach and cook for 2 minutes or until the spinach wilts, stirring occasionally.
4. Remove from the heat and stir in the coconut paste and salt. Serve with a spoonful of rice.

Day 26: Rocket Pizza with Poached Egg

A slightly different take on the traditional pizza. The added egg is a great source of protein without too many extra calories. You can either use the spinach base from Day 7 (see page 211), or you can use a small shop-bought one – either way a really delicious meal.

Ingredients

100 g (4 oz) pizza base, (or use the pizza base recipe from Day 7)
30 g (1 oz) ricotta cheese or cream cheese
50 g (2 oz) grated hard cheese
1 large free-range egg
100 g (4 oz) rocket
Pinch of ground sea salt
Pinch of freshly ground black pepper

Method

1. Preheat oven to pizza base instructions or make the spinach base (see page 211). Turn oven to 160°C /350°F/ Gas 4.
2. In a saucepan, very gently heat the ricotta or cream cheese with the hard cheese to combine, then spread the cheese mixture over the pizza base, leaving a slight uncovered border around the edge. Bake for 5 minutes.
3. As the pizza bakes, poach an egg until medium-hard, or your desired yolk hardness.
4. Top the cooked pizza with rocket and the poached egg, and season to taste. Serve with a baked sweet potato.

Day 27: Blue Cheese Omelette with Rustic Chunky Chips

I really like omelettes, although I have to admit my husband is far better at making them than I am. Getting that lovely soufflé bit under the grill at the very end is essential; it makes the whole meal really great to look at as well as eat.

Ingredients

2 medium potatoes
1 tbsp vegetable oil
¼ tsp celery salt
4 medium free-range eggs
1 tbsp skimmed milk
Pinch of ground sea salt
Pinch of freshly ground black pepper
50 g (2 oz) blue cheese, grated

Method

1. Set the oven temperature to 200°C/425°F/Gas 7.
2. You can cook the rustic chips in two ways:
   - Either cut the potatoes into long chip shapes, rinse under a cold tap and pat dry. Spread on a large non-stick baking tray and toss with a little oil and the celery salt. Lie them flat and roast for 35–45 minutes, turning them a quarter turn now and then, and cook until golden brown and crisp all over.
   - Or cook the coated potatoes in the microwave until just underdone then carefully cut them into long

      chip shapes and either grill or bake in the oven until golden brown.

3. While the rustic chips are cooking, whisk the eggs with the milk, salt and pepper, getting as much air into the mixture as possible.

4. When the chips are ready, cook the beaten eggs in a lightly oiled frying pan.

5. Add the cheese just as the omelette is setting, then place under a very hot grill for 2–3 minutes until the omelette has risen slightly. Serve with the rustic chips immediately.

Day 28: Three-bean Chilli and Rice

Chilli is a great meal all year around, it is really tasty for the whole family and is a great meal for the socialising list too. Serves four.

Ingredients

1 tbsp olive oil
½ medium onion, chopped
1 medium green pepper, chopped
2 garlic cloves, crushed
2 tbsp tomato purée
2 tsp chilli powder
2 tsp ground cumin
¼ tsp ground black pepper
1 can (400 g/14 oz) chickpeas, rinsed and drained
1 can (400 g/14 oz) red kidney beans, rinsed and drained
1 can (400 g/14 oz) black-eyed beans, rinsed and drained
1 can (400 g/14 oz) chopped tomatoes with juice
240 ml (8 fl oz) vegetable stock
1 tbsp ground coriander
100 g (4 oz) sour cream
75 g (3 oz) cooked brown rice (optional)
8 taco trays
Sour cream, to serve

Method

1. Heat the olive oil in a large saucepan over a medium-high heat, add the onion, pepper and garlic to the pan and sauté for 3 minutes.

2. Add 180 ml (6 fl oz) water and the tomato purée, chilli powder, cumin, ground pepper, all the beans, tomatoes, stock and coriander, and bring it all to the boil. Reduce the heat and simmer for 8 minutes.

3. Serve in taco trays with a topping of sour cream and undressed shredded lettuce with a small side dish of brown rice if desired.

Soup Recipes

The following recipes offer a great variety of tasty and satisfying soups, which will help at lunchtime to stop any diet-damaging afternoon grazing. Soups are so versatile flavour-wise, and you can make soup using just about any type of vegetable – fresh, frozen or even canned. Plus they can be 'souper' quick too: I have made a really flavour-packed soup in under five minutes using just frozen veggies and a quick stock. If you do use frozen vegetables like broccoli or cauliflower, just reduce the amount of stock a little to allow for their frozen water content – you can always add a bit more water or stock if needed as you go along. Soups are such a practical and diet-friendly meal – you can make batches of all these soups too and freeze them for later. Adding 200 ml (7 fl oz) of skimmed milk when blended will give a creamier taste. However, if you add the milk do not freeze the soup.

Day 2: Carrot and Coriander Soup with Homemade Croutons

A lovely retro favourite which, with some nice baked croutons for a bit of extra crunch, makes a real lunchtime treat.

Ingredients

1 tbsp vegetable oil
1 small onion, roughly chopped
1 garlic clove, crushed
Pinch of ground sea salt
Pinch of freshly ground black pepper
1.5-2 l (2½–3½ pt) vegetable stock (saving a little for the blending process if needed)
450 g (1 lb) carrots, peeled and roughly sliced
1 tsp ground coriander
1 thick slice stale wholemeal bread
Grating of nutmeg (optional)

Method

1. In a large heavy saucepan, heat the oil on a medium heat then sweat the onion until clear and just browning. Next, add the garlic for a few moments – do not let it burn – and seasoning. Add most of the stock, plus the carrots and coriander and bring it all to the boil. Reduce the heat and simmer until the carrots are tender (around 10 minutes).

2. Remove the pan from the heat and allow the soup to cool for a few minutes.

3. Blend in a food processor or with a hand blender until really smooth – you may need to do this in a couple of batches. Sieve it if you do not have a blender.

4. For the croutons, bake 2.5 cm (1 in) cubes of stale wholemeal bread, the thicker sliced the better, in an oven at 230°C/450°F/Gas 8 for 3–5 minutes until crunchy. You can batch-bake the croutons and keep them in an airtight container for other soups.

5. Serve the soup with the croutons and a little nutmeg sprinkled on top, if desired.

Day 8: Butternut Squash Soup

This a tasty and very satisfying soup, great for the winter months but just as good all year round.

Ingredients

1 small onion, roughly chopped
1 garlic clove, crushed
1 tbsp vegetable oil
½ tsp ground ginger
1.5–2 l (2½–3½ pt) vegetable stock, saving a little for the blending process if needed
½ tsp thyme
Pinch of ground sea salt
Pinch of freshly ground black pepper
1 medium butternut squash, peeled, deseeded and cut into wedges

Method

1. In a large saucepan on a medium heat, sauté the chopped onion and garlic in the vegetable oil, then add the ginger and allow it to infuse with the onion and garlic.
2. Next, add most of the stock, herbs, seasoning and butternut squash. Bring it to the boil, then reduce the heat and simmer until the butternut squash is tender. Remove the pan from the heat and let the soup cool for a few minutes, then blend in a food processor or with a hand blender until smooth. Add a little of the saved stock if you want a slightly less thick soup.

Day 15: Broccoli and Yellow Pepper Soup

This is not only great to taste, but a fabulous-looking soup too. Give it a small swirl of single cream and it is a great starter for dinner parties.

Ingredients

1 tbsp vegetable oil
1 small onion, roughly chopped
1 medium yellow pepper, chopped – frozen pepper is fine to use
½ tsp basil
1.5–2 l (2½–3½ pt) vegetable stock
500 g (1 lb) broccoli, chopped – use all of the broccoli, not just the florets. Frozen broccoli is fine to use
Pinch of ground sea salt
Pinch of freshly ground black pepper

Method

1. Heat the oil in a large saucepan over a medium heat then sauté the onion and pepper with the basil until the onion is just translucent – do not let it burn.
2. Next, add most of the stock and the broccoli and bring to a gentle boil, then reduce the heat and simmer until the broccoli is cooked (about 10 minutes). The broccoli may break up during the simmering, but do not worry as it will all be blended at the end. Season to taste.
3. Remove from the heat and let the soup mixture cool for a few minutes.
4. Blend it all in a food processor or with a hand blender

until really smooth, you may need to do the soup in a couple of batches.

5. Serve with a sprinkling of croutons.

Day 19: Parsnip and Apple Soup

A nice rich and slightly sweet soup which makes a change. For a really quick soup use frozen parsnips and some canned apple.

Ingredients

1 small onion, roughly chopped
1 tbsp vegetable oil
500 g (1 lb) parsnips, peeled and chopped – not too big as they can have a woody texture
Pinch of ground sea salt
Pinch of freshly ground black pepper
½ tsp thyme
1.5–2 l (2½–3½ pt) vegetable stock
1 large cooking apple or 2 medium-sized green eating apples, peeled, cored and chopped
¼ tsp cinnamon

Method

1. In a large saucepan on a medium heat, sauté the chopped onion in the vegetable oil, then add the parsnips, seasoning, thyme and two-thirds of the stock and simmer until just tender.
2. Next, add the chopped apple and the rest of the stock and simmer for a further 5–7 minutes until the apples are starting to break up.
3. Remove the soup from the heat and let it cool down for a few minutes, then blend in a food processor or with a hand blender until smooth. Serve with a pinch of cinnamon on the top.

Day 22: Chilli, Lentil and Tomato Soup

A really great satisfying soup that could easily make a main course if you are ever pushed for time.

Ingredients

1 small onion, roughly chopped
1 garlic clove, crushed
1 tbsp vegetable oil
½ tsp chilli powder
1.5 l (2½ pt) vegetable stock
1 can (400 g/14 oz) chopped tomatoes, drained – keep the
*   juice and add it to the stock*
1 can (400 g/14 oz) green lentils, rinsed and drained
Pinch of ground sea salt
Pinch of freshly ground black pepper

Method

1. In a large saucepan on a medium heat, sauté the chopped onion and garlic in the vegetable oil until softened, then add the chilli powder and stir for 1 minute.
2. Next, add the stock, tomatoes and lentils. Bring to a gentle boil, then simmer for 5 minutes. Season to taste. Remove from the heat and allow to cool before blending.
3. You can either blend it to make a smooth soup, or if you prefer a slightly chunkier texture, quickly pulse in a food blender.

Dessert Recipes

Day 1: Spiced Orange Sorbet

A lovely sharp taste to complete any meal.

Ingredients

300 ml (10 fl oz) orange juice
Pinch of cinnamon
100 g (4 oz) caster sugar
Zest of an orange

Method

1. Put the orange juice, cinnamon and sugar into a medium saucepan. Bring to the boil and keep stirring, until all the sugar has dissolved.
2. Remove from the heat and allow the mixture to cool.
3. Next, pour into a freezerproof container and freeze until firm. Stir every hour or so with a fork to break up the ice crystals. Serve with a sprinkling of grated orange zest.

Day 7: Pineapple and Ginger Compote

A slightly different and quick take on a tasty compote.

Ingredients

1 tbsp Greek yoghurt
1 tbsp fromage fraîs
2 rings of canned pineapple, drained and chopped
2 ginger nut biscuits, crushed
Pinch of ground cinnamon

Method

1. Mix the yoghurt and fromage fraîs together, then stir in the chopped pineapple.
2. Take two individual glass tumblers and sprinkle most of the crushed biscuits in the bottom. Spoon the yoghurt mixture over the ginger nut biscuits, sprinkle the remainder of the biscuits on the top with a pinch of cinnamon.

Day 8: Chocolate Soufflé

A lovely light chocolate treat which is great as a regular pudding, but is also a fantastic dessert for entertaining.

Ingredients:
30 g (1 oz) caster sugar
20 g (¾ oz) plain flour
½ tbsp cocoa powder
¼ tsp vanilla essence
3 tbsp skimmed milk
1 large egg white
1 tsp oil
1 tsp icing sugar

Method
1. Preheat the oven to 180°C/400°F/Gas 6.
2. Combine half of the caster sugar with the flour, cocoa powder, vanilla essence and milk in a small saucepan and place over a medium heat. Keep stirring for 2 minutes until smooth.
3. Remove from the heat and allow to cool for 5 minutes.
4. While the chocolate mix cools, beat the egg white until it forms fairly stiff peaks. Next, gently fold the remaining half of caster sugar into the egg white one spoonful at a time.
5. Then mix together with the cooled chocolate mixture, again a little at a time. Lightly oil two ramekins and spoon in the mixture. Cook for 15 minutes or until the mixture has puffed up and is set.
6. Remove from the oven and cool for a couple of minutes. Just before serving, dust with a little icing sugar.

Day 12: Strawberry, Vanilla and Cherry Compote

A nice colourful dessert that is another great staple for a dinner party.

Ingredients
1 tbsp Greek yoghurt
1 tbsp fromage fraîs
Few drops of vanilla essence
200 g (7 oz) washed and drained cherries (frozen cherries are fine)
6 strawberries, washed and sliced
Sprig of fresh mint

Method
1. Mix the yoghurt, fromage fraîs and vanilla essence together, then stir in the cherries (defrosted if you are using frozen).
2. Spoon into two glass tumblers and serve with the sliced strawberries and mint on top.

Day 14: Chocolate and Ginger Peaches

The ginger complements the peaches really well in this tasty dessert. Serves two.

Ingredients

4 ginger nut biscuits, crushed
25 g (1 oz) brown sugar
2 large ripe peaches, halved and pitted
15 g (½ oz) butter
15 g (½ oz) dark chocolate shavings

Method

1. Combine the crushed biscuits and brown sugar.
2. Hollow out one third of the centre of each peach half with a teaspoon or melon ball maker. Fill each peach half with a rounded tablespoon of biscuit and sugar mixture, pushing it in quite firmly.
3. Arrange peaches in an ovenproof dish, then place 1 level teaspoon of butter on top of each peach half.
4. Place under a medium grill for 2 minutes or until the butter melts. Serve straight away with a sprinkling of shaved chocolate.

Day 16: Mango and Berry Compote

I really like this flavour as the mango complements the slight sharpness of the berries beautifully. Serves two.

Ingredients

3–4 thin slices mango, if using canned rinse before using
1 tbsp Greek yoghurt
1 tbsp fromage frais
100 g (4 oz) mixed berries, either fresh or thawed if frozen

Method

1. Place the slices of mango around the insides of two medium wine glasses.
2. Mix the yoghurt and fromage frais together and spoon over the mango.
3. Place the well-drained berries on top just before serving.

Day 18: Berry Ice-cream Yoghurt with Flaked Almonds

The almonds give a nice crunchy texture to a lovely quick dessert. Eat soon after making as once the berries melt you will end up with a smoothie.

Ingredients

200 g (7 oz) frozen mixed berries – only defrost enough to be able to food-process
5 tbsp Greek yoghurt
1 tbsp clear honey
1 tsp flaked almonds

Method

1. Mix the berries, Greek yoghurt and honey in a food processor for about 20 seconds until it has the consistency of ice-cream.
2. Serve in glass tumblers with a topping of flaked almonds.

Day 23: Apricot and Walnut Compote

A delicious, simple and quick combination of fruit and nuts with the smoothness of fromage fraîs.

Ingredients

1 tbsp Greek yoghurt
1 tbsp fromage fraîs
2–3 fresh or canned apricots, chopped fairly small – rinse if using canned
2 walnuts, chopped

Method

1. Mix the yoghurt, fromage fraîs, apricots and half of the walnuts together.
2. Serve in two glass tumblers with the remaining walnuts as a topping.

Day 25: Apple and Pear Meringue

I have included pear in this one, however the apple goes well with lots of other fruits and the lovely crunchy meringue complements the fruits wonderfully.

Ingredients
1 medium apple, cooking or firm eating
1 medium pear
1 tbsp lemon juice
1 tbsp brown sugar
1 egg white
15 g (½ oz) caster sugar
1 tbsp cocoa powder

Method
1. Preheat the oven to 150°C/325°F/Gas 3.
2. Peel and chop the apple and pear and simmer on a low–medium heat with the lemon juice and brown sugar.
3. While the apple and pear mixture is cooking, whisk the egg white until it forms stiff peaks, then gently fold in the caster sugar and cocoa powder.
4. Spoon the fruit mixture into individual ovenproof bowls and then spread the meringue on top and bake for 10–12 minutes or until firm to touch.

Salad Dressings

These great dressings give a lovely extra taste to any salad, and a little goes a long way. They are all really easy to make and keep in the fridge for a couple of days.

Zesty Yoghurt Salad Dressing

Ingredients
2 tbsp Greek yoghurt
1 tbsp white wine vinegar
½ tsp lemon juice
1 tsp Dijon mustard
1 tsp clear honey
Pinch of ground sea salt
Pinch of freshly ground black pepper
½ tsp lemon zest

Method
1. Whisk the yoghurt, vinegar, lemon juice, mustard and honey together.
2. Stir in the seasoning and the lemon zest. You can keep stored in a sealed container in the fridge for up to two days.

Smooth and Creamy Salad Dressing

Ingredients
1 tbsp mayonnaise
1 tsp clear honey
2 tsp white wine vinegar
½ tsp Dijon mustard (optional)
Pinch of ground sea salt
Pinch of freshly ground black pepper

Method
1. Whisk together all the ingredients.
2. Stir in the seasoning. You can keep stored in a sealed container in the fridge for two days.

Tangy Blue Cheese Salad Dressing

Ingredients

15 g (½ oz) *blue cheese*
2 *tbsp Greek yoghurt*
1 *tbsp mayonnaise*
1 *tsp lemon juice*
1 *tsp white wine vinegar (optional)*
Pinch of ground sea salt
Pinch of freshly ground black pepper

Method

1. Crumble the blue cheese into a bowl and mix in the yoghurt with a fork until smooth.
2. Next, stir in the mayonnaise, lemon juice, vinegar and seasoning. Store in the fridge for up to two days.

Zingy Balsamic Salad Dressing

Ingredients

30 ml (1 fl oz) balsamic vinegar
1 tsp soy sauce
1 tsp wholegrain or Dijon mustard
2 tbsp olive oil

Method

1. Either whisk everything together with a fork or small hand whisk or place all the ingredients in a clean jar, replace the lid tightly and shake vigorously.
2. Use what you need and leave the rest in the fridge for another time; this will store for up to five days.

conclusion

You have done so well to work through the *Stop Overeating* plan and you will now have the understanding and psychological tools you need to do something about your emotional eating once and for all. During the four weekly sessions you have been exploring and investigating all of the factors, situations, places, people and relationships which have led to your emotional eating.

The fact is that there will always be situations and encounters which upset and distress you – as Lucy, the very first person quoted in the book, says, '*I believe it's called life.*' But instead of turning to food to deal with life when it gets upsetting, difficult or boring, you now have lots of different psychological strategies and tactics to help you cope with whatever life tries to throw at you. Note the word **tries** there, because one of the important things you have been learning is that you do not have to accept the issues and problems that others may try to put on you.

Undertaking everything in *Stop Overeating* is a lot to do in one go, so be kind to yourself. If you need a short break, or you are finding it hard to do all at once, this book will always be available to you to pick up again. Over many years of working with clients, I have seen people take a break from their therapy and pick it up again a few weeks or months later. In the meantime they have found it extremely useful to use all the exercises, techniques and strategies they have learnt before returning to carry on and finish everything off.

With all the work you have been undertaking, all the discoveries and observations you have been making about the different situations and people in your life, you now do not always have to be the person who automatically turns to food when they are emotionally provoked. Turning to food has previously been your default reaction, but with all the challenging psychological work you have completed, your default button has been reset. As you continue to react to difficult and distressing situations by choosing not to eat, your power and control over your eating will grow further. Your future health and life choices are being fundamentally changed.

Now you have finished the sessions you will be aware of all the situations and encounters, both in the moment and the long term, that have the potential to emotionally upset or distress you, but crucially you are aware of your potential response to them. Having this awareness and being able to apply the techniques and strategies in the *Stop Overeating* plan, you are now at last in the best psychological position to end your emotional eating. There may have been some areas and subjects you have found difficult to face and deal with – it will always be helpful to go back over a few areas to consolidate what you have learnt; this is quite common in one-to-one therapy.

I hope you have been able to follow the 28-day Eating Plan too. In my experience, people who have got into the habits of eating more healthily for a dedicated period of time have found it easier to carry on applying the *Stop Overeating* techniques, as they have formed a more positive association between healthy food and their emotions.

The *Stop Overeating* tool kit may not work absolutely every time, but even if you have a blip, keep applying what you have learnt and go back over relevant parts of the *Stop Overeating* plan if needed.

Ultimately, you are always going to be your own very best advocate and help, so listen to what you have to say. Remind yourself right now that, through all the hard work you have been undertaking, you are in your best ever position to be able to control any emotional eating and finally lose weight once and for all. Congratulations!

acknowledgements

Thanks must first go to my family, my brilliant husband Steve and wonderful children Joe, Harvey and Elsa, whose support, encouragement and (in some cases) pure bafflement helped to create this book. Thanks also to Abigail Kingston, who gave her welcome and valuable nutritional advice and input.

This is my first book and I have been so very well looked after by everyone at Vermilion, especially Catherine Knight and Susanna Abbott, who saw the vision of my idea and helped me develop and craft it. Thanks to Clare Hulton, my agent, for your much-needed belief and support. Also to all my family, friends and colleagues who have spent a great many meals and countless hours helping me road test my recipes to get them spot on.

The idea for this book came about after many years of providing therapy to several hundreds of clients, with lots of varied and troubling issues. I thank you for sharing your problems, solutions, inspiration and successes with me. As psychologists, we cannot grow and develop without our clients, so thank you.

index

28-day eating plan 7–8, 26, 64, 81, 102, 183–263
  how to use 187–9
  recipes 202–63
  snacks 199–201
  week-by-week menus 189–99
    abandonment and rejection 32, 39, 43, 122, 123–4
acceptance 126
acknowledgement 117, 120, 126–30
  of achievements 81, 200
  and challenging negative emotional messages 144
  and fear of missing out 176
addictions (neurological motivations) 4, 66, 82, 86–7, 89, 90, 91, 103, 173
  case study: Frank 87
adult experiences
  food relationships 72
  food relationships case studies 73–4, 77, 78–9
  personal relationships 54
advocate/s
  envisaged 141–2, 144, 147, 149, 152

self as 36, 62, 171, 180–1, 267
allowance days 5, 155, 156, 178–81
  case study: Chris 178–9
  staying focused 179–81
anxiety/ies 24, 30, 32, 34, 35, 36, 78
  at being caught eating 80
  calming with food 98
  childhood 147
  and fear of missing out 172, 176
  separate therapeutic work on 92
  using food to cope with 79, 88, 96, 98, 112, 113

Backward Step Technique see emotional triggers
beliefs of an emotional eater 4, 66, 91–102, 103, 180
  Beliefs exercise 95–6
  believe in yourself 100–1
  case study: Frank 97–8, 101
  case study: Kate 96–7, 101
  case study: Linda 99–100, 101
  the truth about 93–102

case studies 6–7 *see also*
    individual names or specific
    subjects
challenging negative emotional
    messages 5, 104, 138–54,
    180
  case study: Frank 146–9
  case study: Kate 144–6
  case study: Linda 149–51
  Challenge exercise 140–2
  easy alternative (reverse
    statements) 151–2
  Mini Moment Intervention
    111
  using envisaged advocates
    141–2
childhood
  and food relationships 72
  food relationships cases
    studies 73, 75–6, 77–8
  and formation of self-concept
    53
  insecurity 54, 174, 175
  and origins of fear of missing
    out 174
  and use of food for emotional
    control 75
Chris (case study)
  allowance days 178–9

depression 80
  separate therapeutic work on
    92
dessert recipes 251–9
  apple and pear meringue 259
  apricot and walnut compote
    258

berry ice-cream with flaked
    almonds 257
chocolate and ginger peaches
    255
chocolate soufflé 253
mango and berry compote
    256
pineapple and ginger compote
    252
spiced orange sorbet 251
strawberry, vanilla and cherry
    compote 254
diets and dieting
  difficulties and failures 9, 14,
    67, 81, 83, 93, 95, 101,
    105
  role of emotions 3
  self-support 60, 63
  serial 1, 3, 8, 68
  starvation 188
  successful 2, 80, 84, 90, 138
  see also allowance days; fear
    of missing out; saboteurs;
    28-day plan
dinner recipes 202–42
  blue cheese omelette with
    rustic chunky chips 239–40
  blue cheese polenta with
    sun-dried peppers and
    mushrooms 206–7
  chicken stir-fry 210
  chickpea curry with brown
    rice 237
  chilli steaks and salsa 235
  creamy light macaroni cheese
    with butternut squash
    219–20

creamy mushroom spaghetti 233–4

creamy salmon and broccoli pasta 230

fish and rustic chunky chips 204–5

grilled portobello mushrooms with Wensleydale cheese crumble 217–18

mushroom and thyme risotto 203

pan-fried pork chops and homemade apple sauce 223–4

paprika chicken with asparagus 227

pasta twirls with kale and cheese 213

pasta with sun-dried tomato pesto and feta cheese 225

polenta with sautéed mushroom, courgettes and goat's cheese 228–9

rocket pizza with poached egg 238

root vegetable curry 215–16

salmon spinach with spiced crème fraîche 232

spicy chicken with broccoli 214

spicy root and lentil casserole 226

spinach base margherita pizza 211–12

stuffed cheesy peppers 221–2

tagliolini with almond pesto 202

three-bean chilli and rice 241–2

warm gemelli with cherry tomato and artichoke salad 236

winter vegetable casserole with herb dumplings 208–9

zesty yoghurt Greek lamb chops with aubergine and courgette grills 231

eating habits *see* habits

embarrassment about self-reflection 119

Emotion Identification *see* experienced emotions

emotional chain of events 80, 88, 104, 106

effects of not analysing 118–19

understanding (session1/week 1) 4, 9–26, 65, 93, 103, 174, 180

emotional chain of events analysis

and Mini Moment Interventions 111

and self-sabotage 170

emotional triggers 2, 9, 12–26, 43, 65, 106

Backward Step Technique 11, 14–15, 16–26, 30, 93, 123, 143

Backward Step Technique instructions 16–18

broken allowance day promises as 179

case study: Frank 21–2, 25

case study: Kate 18–20, 25, 44

case study: Linda 22–4, 25

fear of failure as 100

food and eating as 69, 80, 85

experiencing high number 120

and here and now eating 105

identifying 10, 13–14

making notes about 118

psychological links to experienced emotions 27

your flight of stairs 15–16

emotional waves 108–9, 113, 130–1

emotions

associations with food 75

role in weight-loss success 3

separating from food 2

see also experienced emotions

experienced emotions 9, 10, 27–36, 65

Emotion Identification 11, 29–36, 39, 41

Emotion Identification instructions 29–30

case study: Frank 34, 44

case study: Hannah 27, 28–9

case study: Kate 32–3, 44

case study: Linda 35–6, 45

identifying and exploring emotions 27–9

list 31

and negative emotional messages 28–9, 37–8

recalling and tolerating 133

see also emotional waves

'fake it until you make it' approach 142

family relationships 15, 52–4, 56

fear and concerns about trying to stop emotionally eating 95

case study: Linda 99–100, 101

fear of missing out (FOMO) 5, 155, 156, 172–7

case study: Helena 172, 173

planning ahead 176–7

psychological origins 173–4

and social eating 174–6

five Ws (What, Where, When, Who, Why) 72, 110

food

addictions 4, 66, 82, 86–7, 89, 90, 91, 103, 173

association with emotions 75

as comfort 6, 7, 44, 74, 75, 10, 37, 39, 54, 55, 66, 111, 122

as a coping mechanism 26, 36, 47, 54, 66–7

as emotional compensation 77, 175

as emotional trigger 80, 85

habits 2, 4, 66, 82, 83–6, 90, 91, 103

high-calorie, high-fat 1–2, 83–4, 172–3

pre-occupation with 4, 66, 82, 88–90, 90, 91, 103
as punishment 7, 10, 37, 54, 55, 66, 105–6, 111
as suppressor 6, 45, 7, 10, 37, 54, 55, 66, 77, 111
see also relationship with food
food associations 70–1
food history 71–2
forgiveness 126
Frank (case study) 12, 66
addictions 87
Backward Step Technique 21–2, 25
beliefs about being an emotional eater 97–8, 101
challenging negative emotional messages 146–9, 151, 152
Emotion Identification 44
Maxi Effect Analysis 117, 128–30
Mini Moment Intervention 114–15
Real Food Relationships 75–7
Relationship Analysis 60–1
saboteurs 165
secondary gains 97–8, 101
Statement of Feelings 44–5
as suppressor 6, 45, 77
use of food as emotional compensation 175
fruit 184
list and portion sizes 184–5

Graham (case study)
planning to emotionally eat 106–7

habits 2, 4, 66, 82, 83–6, 90, 91, 103
case study: Kate 84–5
getting out of one into another 183–4
Hannah (case study)
experienced emotions 27, 28–9
Helena (case study)
fear of missing out 172, 173
herbs 201

identity as an emotional eater 94, 122
case study: Kate 96–7, 101, 122
in-the-moment emotional eating 103–4, 105, 107, 108

Justine (case study)
saboteurs 168

Kate 12, 66, 175
Backward Step Technique 18–20, 25, 44
beliefs about being an emotional eater 96–7, 101
challenging negative emotional messages 144–6, 151, 152
as comforter 6, 7, 39, 44, 74, 122
Emotion Identification 32–3, 39, 44

habits 84–5
identity as an emotional eater
96–7, 101, 122
Maxi Effect Analysis 117
Mini Moment Intervention
111–14
Real Food Relationships 73–5
Relationship Analysis 59–60
saboteurs 163–4
Statement of Feelings 42,
43–4
themes 123–5
knowledge and power 90

learnt subconscious reactions
28–9
Leave It types 161
Linda 12, 66, 175
Backward Step Technique
22–4, 25
beliefs about being an
emotional eater 99–100,
101
challenging negative
emotional messages 149–
51, 152
Emotion Identification 35–6,
45
fear and concerns about
trying to stop emotional
eating 99–100, 101
Maxi Effect Analysis 118,
124–6
Mini Moment Intervention
115
pre-occupations with food
88–9

as punishment 7
Real Food Relationships
77–80
Relationship Analysis 61–2
saboteurs 166–7
Statement of Feelings 45–6

Maxi Effect Analysis 104,
117–37, 180
acknowledgements 117, 120,
126–30
case study: Frank 117,
128–30
case study: Linda 118, 124–6
case study: Kate 117
exploring self-sabotage 170
instructions 119–20
themes 117, 120, 122–6
tolerating 118, 120, 130–6
understanding the best thing
to do 118–19
Me and Food, What
Happened? (session 2/week
2) 4, 65–102
Mini Moment Intervention
103–4, 105–16, 117, 125,
131, 141, 180
case study: Frank 114–15
case study: Kate 111–14
case study: Linda 115
emotional waves 108–9, 113
and fear of missing out 176
in-the-moment emotional
eating 103–4, 105, 107,
108
instructions 109–11
making notes 110, 118

planning to emotionally eat
105–7, 1–8
stopping allowance days
179–80
stopping self-sabotage 170
Moving Beyond Emotional
Eating (session 4/week 4) 5,
155–81

negative emotional messages 9,
37–47, 63–4, 65
acceptance rooted in survival
technique 149
activated by experienced
emotions 28–9, 37–8
case study: Frank 44–5
case study: Kate 42, 43–4
case study: Linda 45–6
emotional overeating as
response to 10, 13–14, 28,
66–7, 88
and the fear of failure 100
here and now eating response
105
limiting to three statements
43–4
playground bully analogy
54–5
reluctance to confront 46–7
Statement of Feelings 11,
38–9, 40, 41–6, 140
Statement of Feelings
instructions 41–2
storing up, and planning
emotional eating 105
tolerating 118, 130–6
uniqueness 39–40

see also challenging negative
emotional messages
negative internalisation 107

oven temperatures 201

Paul (case study)
relationship legacy 57–8
planning to emotionally eat
105–7, 108
case study: Graham 106–7
playground example 54–5
positive attributes
introducing into internal
dialogue 33
list 153–4
and reversed statements
151–3
pre-occupations with food 4,
66, 82, 88–90, 90, 91,
103
case study: Linda 88–9
psychological aspects of
overweight 3
psychological change
facilitating 121
importance of 56, 130
and others' inflexibilities 63
resistance to 130, 140
psychological containment 43,
47, 121
psychological tools 5, 8, 86,
177, 180

recipes see dessert recipes;
dinner recipes; salad
dressings; soup recipes

relationship with food 4, 65–6,
    68–81, 91, 103
  case study: Frank 75–7
  case study: Kate 73–5
  case study: Linda 77–80
  case study: Miriam 68–9
  and childhood insecurity
    174
  and the FOMO moment 173
  Real Food Relationships 70,
    71, 72–81
  Real Food Relationships
    instructions 72–3
relationships 10–11, 15, 37,
    47–63, 64, 65, 180
  acknowledging treatment by
    others 126–30
  case study: Frank 60–1
  case study: Kate 59–60
  case study: Linda 61–2
  case study: Paul 51–2
  effect on self-concept and
    self-esteem 48, 49, 123
  family 15, 49, 52–4
  legacy 48–53
  power of 54–6
  Relationship Analysis 56–63,
    123, 141
  Relationships Analysis
    instructions 57–8
  romantic 49
  social 49
  two layers 48
  work 48
reflection 62, 82, 89, 136–7
responsibility
  identifying others' 143

  taking on too much 46, 91–2,
    99
rewards, non-food 200
romantic relationships 49

saboteurs 5, 155–6, 157–71
  case study: Frank 165
  case study: Justine 157–8,
    160, 168
  case study: Kate 163–4
  case study: Linda 166–7
  don't get paranoid 170
  ignorant 161, 164, 167,
    168–9
  jealous 160
  sceptical 161–2, 166
  superior 162–3
  tips 168–9
  use of surprise by 168
  see also self-sabotage
salad dressings 260–3
  smooth and creamy salad
    dressing 261
  tangy blue cheese salad
    dressing 262
  zesty yoghurt salad dressing
    260
  zingy balsamic vinegar salad
    dressing 263
secondary gains 94, 130, 143
  case study: Frank 97–8,
    101
self-affirmation 152–3
self-awareness 180–1, 266
self-blame 68
self-compassion 47, 81, 119,
    132

self-concept 49–50
  awareness of external factors
    affecting 14
  based in relationships 48, 49,
    123
  and beliefs about others'
    feelings 48
  formation 53
  'I'm unlovable' 50
  modest shift in 143, 152
  and negative emotional
    messages 38, 45, 54–5, 64,
    137, 138
  preventing further damage
    136
  saboteurs' 158–9, 167
  undermining by planned
    emotional eating 105,
    106–7
  understanding who and what
    is causing fragility 120–1
  and your real self 24–5
self-esteem
  damaging through planning
    to emotionally eat 105, 107
  damaged by negative
    emotional messages 139
  identifying who or what is
    causing low 120–1, 123
  improving 143
  and self-concept 50
self-perception
  overcoming negative 40
  overeating risks of negative
    49
  possibility of change 56
self-reliance 60, 62, 63

self-sabotage 98, 165, 166,
  170–1
shame 91–2
snacks 199–201
  in front of TV 183–4
  list of healthy 201
  quantity and quality 199
social relationships 49
social situations 174–6
  planning ahead 176–7
soup recipes 243–50
  broccoli and yellow pepper
    soup 247–8
  butternut squash soup 246
  carrot and coriander soup
    with homemade croutons
    244–5
  chilli, lentil and tomato soup
    250
  parsnip and apple soup
    249
  recipe tips 243
Start to Stop (session 3/week 3)
  5, 14, 103–54
Statement of Feelings *see*
  negative emotional
  messages

Take It types 161, 169, 176
teenagers/adolescents
  and food relationships 72
  food relationships case
    studies 73, 76, 77–8
  personal experiences 54
themes 116, 117, 120, 122–6
  case study: Kate 123–5
  in emotional responses 34

from Backward Step
    Technique 22
specific foods 125–6
specific people or types of
    people 123
specific times and situations
    125
therapy 2–3
    and beliefs about being an
        emotional eater 92–3
    meanings of toleration in
        131–2
    reflection during non-therapy
        time 136–7
    repeated people, situations
        and scenarios 121
    replicating one-to-one 2–3, 4,
        5, 11, 30, 66, 71, 82, 89,
        104, 117
    separating out issues 92
    and shame 91–2

therapy exercises 5–6
    emotional and psychological
        challenge 6, 32, 40, 45
    importance of honesty 58–9
    undertaking all in one go for
        each session 11
tolerating 118, 120, 130–6

Understanding the Emotional
    Chain Of Events *see*
    emotional chain of events
uniqueness of emotional eating
    episodes 39–40, 146

vegetables 185
    colour 185
    list and portion sizes 186

weekends 125
work pressures 15
work relationships 48